Locker Room Angels

Evie Kalvelage

TABLE OF CONTENTS

Endorsements

This book is a must-read for any family going through the frightening experience of a bone marrow transplant for their loved one. The author, my sister-in-law, describes how fear can be overcome with knowledge, and with the support of friends, family, strangers, and faith. Her explanations of the medical procedures and complications are succinct and understandable, which as a physician, I know will be very helpful and comforting to the reader. I highly recommend this book.

Kay Watnick MD

Imagine a person you love in a life or death situation. You are his anchor. He was yours. Now, suddenly, he is unmoored and his life depends on trusting physicians, taking risks with alternative treatments, soldiering through abhorrent side effects, and maintaining a positive attitude. But primarily his life depends on you, your steadiness, your faith, your intuition, your resilience.

Locker Room Angels vividly captures the stress, wonder, chaos, miracles, grief, joy, and constant change that occur during an illness. Evie Kalvelage plunges the reader into her true story, using an authentic voice that makes her situation all too universal. The reader easily identifies with the questions, worry, vulnerability, and sorrow she is living through. We are amazed at her and her husband's humor, indomitable spirit, and ability to persevere. This riveting love story is filled with hope and unlikely angels, some who happen to wear sweaty hockey jerseys.

Deborah Shouse, author of Love in the Land of Dementia: Finding Hope in the Caregiver's Journey

If your spouse has cancer or another life-threatening illness, you are not alone. Locker Room Angels takes you on Evie Kavelage's journey from her husband's diagnosis, through successful treatment, and beyond. Let her frank and honest account accompany you as you travel your own road.

Mary-Lane Kamberg, professional writer, editor, and speaker. Writes nonfiction, short fiction, poetry and magazine articles for adults and children. Co-leader of the Kansas City Writers Group

Prologue

"We heard about Doug's situation and we want to do something. I'll be in touch after the teams meet. Hockey guys stick together."

What a surprise—an email from Lutzie, the commissioner of Doug's old-timer's hockey league. I wondered how he knew my Gmail address. This was the first of many email exchanges and phone calls with my Locker Room Angels. They brought intrigue, joy, and gratitude to a time of fear, worry, and uncertainty.

€€€

Doug and I were married for thirteen years—after a 5-year courtship. Our marriage was the second for both of us. I had four children—Jason, Jill, Joel, and Jamie. I suspect that was the reason for our long engagement. Doug had one daughter—Katey. When we married, they became our children.

During that time, Doug trudged to the hockey rink late every Thursday night. He hauled an elephant-sized equipment bag that smelled as if something had crawled in and died. With the devotion of mail carriers, this conglomeration of old-timers pursued their hockey passion in the dead of winter and the heat of summer. For the most part, the game and the tailgating that followed were women-free zones. The team's fan base consisted of a couple of girlfriends once in a while, never wives, and occasionally someone who wandered into the rink by accident.

Doug prided himself on being labeled the fastest guy on the ice. When his league could not get enough old guys, they'd recruit younger players to fill out the roster. After the helmets were off, the subs stared at Doug, and shook their heads. "No way, I can't believe a senior citizen like you beat me down the ice."

Maintaining that reputation exacted a price. Doug often arrived home barely able to drag himself and his bag through the front door. To stay at the top of his game, he walked, lifted weights, and rode his bike up steep hills. He also rollerbladed, dragging a weighted sled, which he invented. The "PAVESLED" used brushes to provide resistance over pavement, similar to football players dragging sleds across a field.

Though I had met a few of Doug's teammates briefly, my images of them emerged primarily from the stories my husband told me. I concluded it would be difficult to tell the difference between their locker room and one in a high school, especially if you closed your eyes against the gray hair and wrinkles. Raunchy jokes and merciless teasing were just as important as chasing the puck.

I appreciated them for the crazy characters they were, but nothing prepared me for how much more there was to these guys. Their friendships ran deep, and their unspoken bonds were sacred.

Our Reprieve is Over

On the way home from work one November day, my cell phone rang. I smiled, hoping it was my husband calling to ask me out to dinner.

"Hey, is our insurance info the same? I don't have my card with me."

"Yeah. Why? What's wrong? Where are you?" My mind jumped to panic mode.

"I'm at the doctor's office. Just getting a few tests."

"Oh my gosh! You never go to the doctor. I'll be there in less than 10 minutes."

I pulled into the parking lot as Doug pushed through the outside doors of the medical office building. His head was bowed, his face pale, and his John Wayne gait absent. I parked and jumped out.

"What's wrong? Why did you go to the doctor?"

"Chill, I'm okay. They checked my lungs. It took two x-rays 'cause they're so big and healthy." He grinned. "My heart checked out too, but I need to get blood drawn." His grin faded.

I put my hand through his arm, and we hustled toward Lab One, a block from the doctor's office. His silence chilled me more than the smell of winter and the cold November wind that whipped my hair in my face. I turned to Doug, gave him a little shove, and stomped my foot on the sidewalk.

"Talk to me. What's wrong?"

He stopped, his shoulders slumped. "Last night when I skated down the ice, I couldn't breathe when I got to the other end. I felt like I was suffocating. It really scared me."

"Oh no!" I grabbed his arm.

"I thought I was gonna' collapse. Finally caught my breath, changed and came home."

The sign in Lab One's window said CLOSED. Doug walked closer and checked the hours. "They open at 7am. I'll come back first thing in the morning."

Daylight was fading as we walked back toward our cars. I shook my head. "I just can't believe you didn't tell me about this."

"It was late. You were already asleep. Didn't wanna bother you. You're such a worrier."

I put my hands on my hips and glared at him.

"Why are you so mad?" He jabbed his upturned hands toward me.

"You didn't say anything before you left for work. Why didn't you tell me you made a doctor's appointment?"

"I guess I should have." He shrugged and tilted his head. "Hey, I was feeling fine, so why get you all revved up?"

"Oh Doug, we were afraid this would happen."

"C'mon, let's go. I'm freezing, and the smell from Master Wok reminds me how hungry I am."

"I'm starving too, but Chinese doesn't sound good. Can we go to Olive Garden?"

"Sure, especially if that'll get me out of the doghouse." He grabbed my hand and walked me to my car.

€€€

As I slid behind the wheel, my thoughts bounced back two years—our first indication something was wrong. Doug's two sisters and I badgered him to get a physical. At sixty, he needed a checkup to establish some baselines. He finally made an appointment.

A few days after his visit, our primary care physician called with unsettling news. Doug's routine blood tests came back with several abnormalities. The doctor referred him to a cancer specialist.

I accompanied him to the appointment. In the waiting room, we looked around uncomfortably. The room was quiet. A couple held hands and whispered in a corner. A young woman, bald from chemo, wore a colorful scarf tied in back. She stared at her Styrofoam coffee cup. Some people dozed. No one looked at the TV news channel droning bad news. They had enough of their own.

Doug bent down to whisper in my ear as we stood in line to check in. "These poor people. And so many of them. We don't belong here."

The receptionist smiled a cheery greeting. "Good morning. Sign in here and the nurse will be with you shortly."

The patients ahead of us returned weak hellos and nods. Doug signed in and we sat near an older man in a wheelchair. I turned to acknowledge him, but his head drooped on his chest. He appeared to be sleeping. Too disturbed to flip through magazines, Doug and I sat silently, occasionally glancing at each other.

A nurse called Doug's name. We gathered our belongings and followed her to an exam room. Shortly after we sat down, Doctor Osgood knocked on the door and entered. He greeted us with a warm handshake, settled himself on the wheeled stool, and rolled close to us. His concerned half smile warned me this wasn't going to be an everything's okay visit.

"How are you feeling?

"Fine. I'm only here 'cause my doc sent me."

"That's very surprising. Your blood test shows you have myelodysplastic syndrome, specifically refractory anemia with excess blasts. RAEB. I know that doesn't make much sense to you, but it's serious. You'll probably want to look it up online."

I had no idea what that meant, but at least the doctor hadn't said the word cancer. Maybe Doug could just take a bunch of iron and get rid of the anemia. That was the only word I recognized.

Doctor Osgood leaned forward, put his elbows on his knees, and folded his hands. "Your fitness has apparently allowed you to cope with your symptoms. Your blood test results would have sent most men your age, even someone much younger, to the couch with a remote."

I looked at Doug. He smiled, proud that his hard work was evident. My stomach churned. My palms were sweaty.

"As long as you're asymptomatic, we'll just monitor your condition. But there's a high probability the disease will worsen. There are treatments to help, but the only real possibility for cure is a bone marrow transplant."

His words hung in the air. I had no clue what was involved, but it sounded deadly serious and frightening. I focused on the fact it offered hope. Doug pressed for more information, but the doctor told us to take it step-by-step. Now was not the time to take that leap.

"Call the scheduler to make a follow-up appointment for two weeks from today. Be sure to come in if you have any new symptoms." The doctor looked back at us with a sympathetic smile. He opened the door and walked out.

Two weeks came and went. Doug felt fine and never made that call. I pretended to forget and didn't remind him. We buried ourselves in denial. He persisted with his exercise regime and weekly hockey.

"Doug, are you feeling okay?" I asked now and then.

"Sure. Why?"

He looked paler and tired more easily, but oh well—he was getting older. He still ran circles around me and all of our friends.

€€€

I pulled into the parking lot at Olive Garden and was jolted to the present. How did I get here? I was so deep into my brooding, I didn't remember driving. It's amazing what we can do on autopilot. The knot in my stomach made me wonder if I could eat—a rare concern for me. Our reprieve was over. The recent episode on the ice eliminated the option of hiding our heads in the sand any longer.

Thankfully, the restaurant wasn't crowded. I found Doug seated in a booth studying the menu. I sat across from him. "Doug, we have to follow up on this."

"I know. I'll go. But I don't feel bad now. I hate to make a big deal out of this. It's probably just a one-time thing. I sure hope it isn't what my dad had."

"Do you think it is? What made you say that?" I leaned forward and stared into his eyes.

"Well, you know Dad had problems with his blood. He had some kind of anemia and my uncle died of leukemia."

"Oh honey, could this be hereditary?" I wrung my hands. "I knew your dad ended up having transfusions several times a week before he passed, but I didn't really understand what was going on. He never complained, and he was so active for an eighty-year-old. I never thought of him as sick."

"I didn't either. Mom said he went to his office every day. He called me every Wednesday to report on his tennis game the night before. Never missed a morning at The Elbow Room for breakfast with his buddies."

"Why didn't we pay more attention? Maybe you should call your mom and get some answers."

"It's hard to keep up when we live fourteen hours away. We only saw him a couple of times a year and he never talked about it. Let's not get carried away. I don't want to bother my mom with this yet. There isn't much to go on. Let's order. I'm starving."

"Okay, but you have to promise me you'll make an appointment and keep it—no matter how you feel."

"Yes Ma'am!" He saluted me.

Dead End... Time to Pivot

On our return visit to the oncologist's office, I had the sinking feeling we belonged here this time. Quiet people whose lives had been drastically altered again filled the waiting room. Jerked from their routine lives, they faced an unexpected future, struggling to survive. At least this place offered a possible second chance.

Were we really part of this group? It seemed surreal. We were both relatively young and Doug was extremely active and healthy. We enjoyed traveling, hiking, golf, tennis and playing with our ten grandkids. Doug rode bikes with them, took them ice-skating, and pushed them tirelessly on the swings hanging from the big oak tree in our front yard. He was the fun Papa who told tall tales. What was to become of our retirement dreams? We were sitting in a cancer clinic.

A nurse led us to an exam room. "The doctor will be in soon." She turned and left, closing the door behind her.

As I sat next to Doug, I noticed there was no exam table.

"I guess this'll just be a consultation. The nurse didn't even take your vitals, and there are only two chairs and a stool."

"Is that bad?" Doug jumped up and paced the small room. Like an unruly two-year-old, he opened every drawer and cabinet.

"I don't know, but can you please sit down? It'll be embarrassing if the doctor walks in."

"What? I'm not doing anything wrong."

I rolled my eyes and shut up.

It wasn't long until Doctor Osgood knocked and walked in, glancing at Doug's chart.

"Sounds like you had a bad episode recently. What's going on?"

Doug described what had happened the last time he played hockey.

"Looks like it's time for further testing. Haven't seen you in a while. I expected to follow up with you sooner."

"Well, I was feeling pretty good until..."

"I understand. When we're finished talking, I'll send the nurse in to draw blood. We'll call you when we get the results. Depending on what we find, there may be a few interim treatments to try, but at best they're temporary."

"Do you think this is hereditary?" Doug squirmed in his seat.

"Why do you ask?"

"Maybe I have what my dad had. He had problems with his blood for years. Before he died, he was getting transfusions a couple times a week. What did you call this?"

"Myelodysplastic syndrome."

"Yup, I'm pretty sure that's what he had."

"It's tempting to assume that, but no testing has conclusively proved this condition is inherited. It does sometimes happen to several people in a family, but that can be due to environmental or other factors."

"One of my uncles died of leukemia. Is that related?"

"This syndrome can evolve into leukemia. Yes."

"It seems likely it could be genetic given that two of Doug's relatives have the same problem." I said. "I'm wondering if Doug's daughter should get checked out."

"I understand why you would think that. Maybe future testing will reveal a link. Right now, here's a good way of thinking about it. If several members of a family are killed in a drive-by shooting, it certainly isn't hereditary." He closed Doug's chart. "The nurse will be in to draw blood, and we'll call you to set up an appointment as soon as we get the results." He shook Doug's hand. "Take care. See you soon."

After the doctor left, Doug and I looked at each other. "I like this guy and he seems to know his stuff, but the odds seem to point to something genetic. That drive-by shooting example made no sense to me. It seems too coincidental that my dad and his brothers...."

"What do you mean brothers?"

"I'm pretty sure my other uncle had the same thing."

"Oh gosh. I agree. The drive-by shooting doesn't make sense to me either. I guess it doesn't matter anyway." I started to stand, then sat. "Oh, we have to wait til they draw blood."

"Wouldn't wanna miss that. I sure hope this girl knows what she's doing. I hate it when they miss and have to stab me more than once."

"I wonder how long it takes to get the results."

€€€

A couple of days later, the office called. Doug made an appointment for early the next week. Back in the exam room that was becoming too familiar, we didn't have to wait long for the doctor. He wasn't smiling.

Doctor Osgood put his hand on Doug's shoulder. "Unfortunately, your results indicate that none of the interim treatments will work for you. I can't do anything more. It's time to see the University of Kansas Bone Marrow Transplant team. I'll set up the appointment."

I slumped in the chair. The first unknown was no longer a mystery. Doug had to have a bone marrow transplant—whatever that meant. Doug bowed his head slightly and didn't say a word. Then he stood and shook the doctor's hand. "Thanks for everything, Doc."

I started to follow my husband out the door. The doctor touched my shoulder. I hesitated and turned around "You'll have to be very strong for Doug."

A chill ran through me. Doctor Osgood's words sounded ominous. They proved to be prophetic.

First Steps

We started the New Year with the big question answered, but it spawned a million new ones. Doug stopped playing hockey and rested more, but he redoubled his efforts to stay in shape as his energy allowed. We both worked full time, gave our best effort to living a normal life, and spent as much time as possible with the grandkids. The uncertainty of the next weeks and months weighed heavily on our minds. We bounced between impatience to get started and trepidation about what the future would bring.

Doug's younger sisters, Kay and Gin, chomped at the bit waiting to be screened as potential matches for the transplant. They called often to check on Doug and fought over who would be the donor if they were both candidates.

Neither of them expressed any concerns or fears about their own health, but all medical procedures have risks. Gin is a nurse and Kay is a doctor. Given their medical background, I'm guessing they researched the process thoroughly. They must have experienced some secret misgivings.

Doug and I studied the process as well. Years ago, bone marrow transplant required surgery and anesthesia—far greater risk and pain for the donor. Today the medical world knows blood-forming cells found in bone marrow are also present in circulating or peripheral blood. This method employs a non-surgical procedure and is used ninety percent of the time. Doug and I were grateful that pain and downtime for the donor was minimal compared to what it used to be.

For five days leading up to the donation, the donor receives injections of filgrastim, a medication to increase the number of blood-forming cells in the bloodstream. It can cause side effects, such as bone pain, muscle aches, headache, fatigue, nausea, and vomiting. These usually disappear within a couple of days after the injections are discontinued.

A catheter—thin, plastic tube—is placed in a vein of the donor's arm. During the process, the donor might feel lightheaded or have chills, numbness or tingling around the mouth, and cramping in their hands. These symptoms go away after the donation. Blood removed through the catheter goes to an apheresis machine that takes out the stem cells. The rest of the blood is returned to the donor through a vein in the other arm. It takes two to six hours as an outpatient procedure. Typically, two to four apheresis sessions are required, depending on how many blood stem cells are collected each time.

According to what we learned, Doug's benefactor would most likely experience some short-lived pain or flu-like symptoms from the injections of filgrastim. After the procedure, most people experience some fatigue. But they are able to resume their normal activities in a few days to a week.

Given the travel inconvenience and possible physical side effects, his sisters would experience an interruption of their busy lives if they were matches. Gin lives in Hawaii. Kay has a dermatology practice in Michigan. Every time we spoke with them, we expressed our deep gratitude for their willingness to go through the process.

Years earlier, Kay's husband, Rick, had been a stem cell donor for his brother who didn't make it. We never discussed that possibility, though I'm sure it lurked in the back of everyone's mind. Despite that history, Doug's sisters were excited and optimistic. Their frequent phone calls helped keep us positive.

We asked the doctors if Katey, Doug's only child could be a match. They informed us that sons and daughters were rarely able to donate. We focused our hope on Gin or Kay. Just in case, the clinic researched the other option, unrelated donors. We continued to study up on the process.

We learned doctors choose ninety-five per cent of donors from the age range between eighteen and forty-four. Would-be donors over sixty are rarely accepted based on increased health risks for them. The registry does not accept anyone under eighteen because a person must be able to give legal consent. Since donation is a voluntary procedure, a parent or guardian cannot give permission. Siblings are an exception to those age ranges.

While we were in limbo, our daughter, Jill, called me. "Mom, I talked to lots of my friends and in-laws. I'm happy to donate. They are too. I'd like to coordinate a donor drive if it would help, in case neither of Doug's sisters works out."

"Oh honey, I'm so touched by your offer. I know how busy you are. Let me email the nurse coordinator and get some details. I'll get back to you."

Beth, the nurse in charge of finding a donor, answered my inquiry later that day. "The odds against that effort being successful finding a match for Doug are huge. It's a great idea and I encourage them to donate, but it won't directly benefit Doug."

Jill was disappointed to hear the news.

"I'm so grateful for the thought, honey. Doug is too. Isn't it crazy, you're actually getting close to the outside age range? By the way, Beth thought it was a great idea for you to register. It could be the gift of life for someone, but it won't be Doug."

"Okay, Mom. With all that's going on right now, I'll probably give it up. I'm praying Gin or Kay will be a match. Hang in there. Tell Doug we love him."

€€€

The process for submitting a sample to be tested is quick and easy. All the potential donor has to do is swab their inner cheek and send it to a lab. A blood sample also works. The test for donors is called HLA or human leukocyte antigen testing. We were surprised to learn the person didn't have to have the same blood type and it didn't matter if it was a man or woman. (Imagine the comments in the Angels' locker room if Doug announced his donor was a woman.) It's all about the HLA protein or marker that's found on most cells in the body. Our immune systems use those markers to identify which cells belong in our bodies and which ones don't.

During this trying time, I was shopping at Walgreens and noticed a sign for Be the Match. It caught my eye only because of what was happening in our lives. How many things like this had I missed because it was off my radar? A small table, manned by a volunteer, held sign-up sheets and kits for recruiting donors. The woman in charge of the campaign was explaining to a curious young man how easy it was.

"You give your consent, wipe the inside of your cheek with the special cotton swab included in this packet, drop the specimen in the pre-addressed envelope, and send it in for testing."

I walked over to the table and touched the man on the arm. "I hate to interrupt, but I wanted to thank you both. My husband needs a bone marrow transplant. We're desperate to find a match in case his sisters don't work out. It means the world to me to see your selfless interest in offering a second chance to a stranger."

€€€

In the middle of January while the search for a donor proceeded, Doug had his first bone marrow biopsy. We sat in the waiting room. My palms were sweaty and my heart raced. A nurse approached us to explain the procedure.

"Doug will lie face down. We'll give him a shot to numb the area. Then we'll use a large hollow needle to aspirate—draw up—a small sample of his bone marrow for evaluation in the lab. Because blood cell components form in the bone marrow, these test results offer doctors more detailed information about the disease than blood drawn from a vein."

Coward that I am, I could not imagine accompanying him into the treatment room. I figured any time you have to get a shot before they stick a needle in you, the second one must be awful. In my mind, the size of the large needle grew to the dimensions of an ice pick.

We waited for a nurse to call Doug's name. At the last minute, I vacillated about going with him. But I didn't change my mind. I stayed in the waiting room with my head down and prayed.

I smelled coffee and looked up to see a volunteer pushing a cart with various drinks and snacks.

"Would you like something to drink or eat?"

"Yes, thank you." Her look of compassion pulled a smile out of me. I grabbed a bottle of water and a small package of Lorna Doone cookies.

I glanced around and noticed the chairs in the large room were full. So many patients and caregivers. So many people hoping to stay alive and even reclaim their health.

"I like your shoes. They look really comfortable," a stylish older woman commented.

"Thank you, they are." A simple compliment began a conversation that kept me busy instead of worried.

I heard Doug come down the hallway before I saw him.

"Next time don't warn me, don't count, just get it over with. I can't believe how brutal you nurses are." He was smiling and so was she.

If you want to deal with Doug, it's imperative to have an expansive sense of humor. Thank heavens, most of the nurses we had encountered did.

She waved. "See you next time."

"Not if I see you first." Doug walked over to me and stood looking down at me. "I'm ready to go."

"Guess it wasn't as bad as we expected. Are you as okay as you seem?" I smiled up at him.

"I'm fine. Let's get out of here."

He seemed to have used up all his good humor with the nurse. I grabbed my purse and book. "Let me have the keys. The nurse said I should drive."

"No, I can drive. It hurt like hell when she jabbed that giant needle in my back, but I'm okay now."

"But Doug...."

"I said I can drive. Let's go."

His wrinkled forehead and gritted teeth caused me to back off. Without further protest, I followed him out of the waiting room to the elevators. What is it about driving? He wants to drive even when he's half-dead. It must be a man-thing or maybe it makes him feel independent. I don't get it, but it's important to him. I don't want to add to the losses he's already suffering. I hope I'm doing the right thing.

Doug got behind the wheel and backed out of the parking space. "Forgive me if I was cranky. I just wanted to get outta there."

On the ride home, we joked and laughed, grateful to have that procedure behind us.

"The nurses sat me at the edge of the exam table to make sure I wasn't dizzy. I got up and staggered around. You should've seen their faces."

"Oh Doug, you didn't."

"They thought it was funny once they realized I was kidding around."

I shook my head. "I'm guessing this is only the start of you making your mark with these poor nurses."

"On Thursday, I guess we'll find out a lot more. They should have the results of this test, and be able to tell us what's next." Doug said.

"I feel so crazy. Sometimes it still doesn't seem real and other times it seems all too real."

"I know what you mean. But I'll tell you that darn needle today was very real."

Reality Hits

The day of our appointment at the BMT Clinic arrived. We followed the signs and spotted a wash station at the entrance. Before we could enter the waiting room, we had to wash our hands. A receptionist told us to touch the handicap push pad with our wrist or elbow to keep our hands clean.

Doug and I entered the large room. I noticed the clean antiseptic smell. Posters proclaiming "Clean Hands Save Lives ... It's that Simple," along with anti-bacterial gel dispensers everywhere underlined the seriousness of this place. We were silent as we looked around the jam-packed room. Doug pointed to a relatively uncrowded corner. We drifted toward it as I continued to scan the room. So many frail people. Numerous patients wore masks and stocking caps. Some used walkers while others sat in wheelchairs. My heart pounded, and the lump in my throat made it hard to swallow. Doug sat and stared straight ahead. I didn't want to ask how he was feeling.

A nurse's aide called Doug's name. She smiled as we got up to follow her. We waited while she quickly wiped down our seats with disposable bleach wipes. She led us through a door, and down the hall. "How are you this morning?"

"We're not sure. Pretty nervous I guess." I said.

"Oh, is this your first time here?"

"Uh-huh," Doug said in a quiet voice. "We're here for a consultation. I guess I need a bone marrow transplant, whatever that means."

"The doctors here are first class. KU is the best place to be. We'll take good care of you." She opened the door to an exam room. "Make yourself comfortable. Can I get you anything? Something to drink? A snack?"

"No thanks." Doug and I said simultaneously.

"The doctor will be with you shortly," she said on her way out.

A few minutes later, a doctor knocked and came in. He declined to shake Doug's hand.

"Hi, I'm Doctor Ganguly." His brilliance and energy lit up the small room. This bone marrow transplant expert poked around on his smart phone, and showed us statistics and mortality rates. He didn't pull any punches as he presented a clear, overwhelming, mind-numbing outline of the precarious position Doug's life was in at this moment. The percentages for full recovery were much lower than I wanted to hear.

What? I smiled that insane smile that pops up just before a bout of inappropriate giggling starts because fear and panic make you senseless and out of control. Did he say just over fifty per cent? Only one in two will survive? That can't be.

I looked at Doug. He listened intently. I twisted my wedding ring and focused on the doctor. What was happening to us?

"For many patients, this is a difficult decision, but for you, the choice is simple. A bone marrow transplant or death within a year, maybe less, depending on how quickly the disease progresses. You have no alternatives."

Dead in a year or less? My mind spun. Nauseous, and light-headed, I tried to hide from the "C" word, despite its presence everywhere around me. No! Doug has something similar to cancer, but not cancer. He just needs treatment by the same kind of doctors.

I finally blurted, "Does my husband have cancer?"

"Yes."

That three-lettered word sucker punched me in the stomach and stripped me of my silly rationalizations. Now I knew. Myelodysplastic syndrome, with excess blasts, (RAEB) was cancer. Untreated, it would progress to acute leukemia and kill my husband in a few months. I touched Doug's hand and glanced at him. He didn't respond. His face was still, emotionless, intent on absorbing this horrendous news.

Doctor Ganguly continued his verbal fountain of fast-paced medical information. "The results of the bone marrow biopsy tell us the disease is Stage Two—the perfect time for a transplant. Stage One is too early for the risk involved. Stages Three and Four make it much more complicated."

Perfect time? Does he mean now? What risks? More complicated?

He wasn't insensitive, but there was no sugarcoating. "KU is a cutting-edge facility. We have lots of experience and the staff is one of the best you'll find anywhere."

Doug spoke up. "I called the cancer center in Seattle. My sister, who's a doctor, recommended I check out City of Hope in Los Angeles, and MD Anderson in Houston."

"In this day and age of technology, we exchange information with doctors all over the country on a daily basis. We meet often at conferences to stay on top of any new trials and treatments. KU is the place for bone marrow transplants in this region. Our extensive experience, your fitness, and general good health increase your chances for survival several percentage points. Again, it's your only choice if you want a chance at life."

Survival? Only chance at life? This had to be a nightmare. Please let me wake up to our old life.

Doug's voice drifted into my stunned thoughts and brought me back to reality. This definitely was not a bad dream. This was real.

"From what I can see," Doug said, "this is a long road. Living far away from home for several months would turn our lives upside down. I have my own business and my wife has a job."

I wanted to scream and run away, but I amazed myself. I sat there like a mature adult. My best efforts to listen to the doctor were futile. His words could not penetrate my devastated mind. My breaths came quickly. I felt dizzy and faint. Do I need a paper bag to avoid hyperventilating? I couldn't look at Doug.

The doctor stood and walked to the door, startling me to attention. "The nurse will be in shortly to draw blood and make follow-up appointments."

I had to get away. "I'm going downstairs for a cup of coffee. Do you want anything?"

"No." Doug answered without looking at me.

I made a quick getaway before tears started.

In the cafeteria, I sat at a table in the corner and looked at smiling, laughing people going about their business. My world had just been shattered. How could everyone and everything around me look normal? The lyrics to The End of the World whirled through my mind. The words fit except it was lost health instead of lost love.

I punched my best friend's number into my cell. "Linda! Doug has cancer. I'm sitting in a lounge at the KU Cancer Clinic. I can count the word cancer twenty times just glancing around. The signs feel like they're screaming at me. 'Cancer Center' 'Do you Love Someone with Cancer?' 'Living with Cancer', 'Fighting Cancer', 'Surviving Cancer.' On and on. I can't get my mind around it. We don't belong here. This can't be happening. It just doesn't seem real. How can it be?"

"Oh no Evie! My heart breaks for you guys. Try to calm down. It'll be all right. Treatments improve every day." She said all the things a best friend says, and promised we would constantly be in her prayers. "Please call me when things settle down. Let me know what the plan is."

After my meltdown, I felt better. Sharing it with Linda somehow made it more manageable. Maybe her prayers had already begun to help. I drank a little of my coffee, but despite lots of cream and sugar it tasted bitter. My stomach churned, too upset to accommodate coffee or food. I threw my cup in the trash, walked into the ladies' room, and splashed cold water on my face. After some deep breaths, I plastered a shaky smile on my face, and took the elevator back up to the BMT clinic on the third floor.

I opened the door to Doug's room. A nurse was smiling and chatting with Doug while she prepared to draw blood. She placed at least twenty test tubes on the table beside him.

"Are you going to take it all? I don't think I have enough to fill those." Miraculously, Doug was in a silly mood.

"I can see you're gonna be a favorite around here." She patted his shoulder and continued her vampire work.

My mood brightened. I straightened up and forced panic and tears away for later. How could Doug cope so well? Hadn't it sunk in yet? Things are actually okay in this moment. I willed myself not to think too far ahead. Isn't that a lesson from many of the devotions I read each morning? Live one day at a time. Tomorrow is God's mystery.

Everyone we'd met here seemed competent, caring, and light-hearted. We faced the fight of our lives—literally. The road ahead would be long and perilous, but it looked as if we had come to the right place.

Hope, Disappointment and Waiting

After the nurse left with half of Doug's blood, Beth, the specialist for matching donors and patients, spoke with us. She was pleased to hear Doug had two sisters who were willing to be donors, especially when we told her Gin, the youngest, was already on the Bone Marrow Registry.

"I'll check on that and get back to you in less than a week," Beth said.

"Kay, Doug's other sister, sent off a sample as soon as we told her he needed a transplant.

"That's great. Hopefully one of them will be a match."

True to her word, Beth emailed us as soon as she found out. Gin was not a match. Frustrated and upset, we kept hope alive that Kay would be the perfect match. In the meantime, I prayed for peace and patience, qualities that became mainstay prayer requests.

A couple of days later, we found out Kay wasn't a match either. We were disappointed and discouraged. The easy solution was not to be. A related donor was the first choice, because it eliminated the need to search Be the Match Bone Marrow Registry. A related donor would save lots of time, effort, and money.

Though she didn't go into detail, Beth assured us a non-related donor was in some respects better than a related donor. The pros and cons balanced each other. She expressed optimism a donor would be found. Given Doug's Caucasian, European ancestry, the odds were excellent.

For American Indian, Alaskan Native, Asian, Black, Hispanic, Native Hawaiian, or Pacific Islander patients, it is much more difficult to find an unrelated match. The registries are always looking for donors from these groups and for multiple racial or ethnic background benefactors.

While the search for the donor continued, Doug had a second bone marrow biopsy. Those results revealed Doug's condition was worsening. While we waited, he would have to take some low dose chemotherapy.

Fortunately, Doctor Osgood's office on our side of town could provide this treatment. Doug would receive Vidaza intravenously (IV) daily, Monday through Friday, for one week, alternating with three weeks off. That schedule would repeat for six months or until the donor was found. At least now, we had a plan. We hoped this bridge to the final treatment would be short.

In early February, my husband, who rarely took even an aspirin, received his first dose of chemo. The administering nurse advised us, "Very few clients have any bad side effects with Vidaza."

Doug and I sat in a room full of recliners and IV poles with a dozen other patients, caregivers, and nurses. Familiar conversations between some of the nurses and patients testified to how much time they had spent together. Some conversed casually as if out for coffee. A few were on their phones while others slept huddled under blankets. They looked weak and puny. How could they even walk out of this treatment room?

I bounced my toes on the ground and looked around, too nervous to knit or read. I averted my eyes from the IV needles and lines that adorned so many arms in that room—especially Doug's. As usual, he was quiet. His solemn demeanor, closed eyes, and quick answers to my unwelcome questions revealed his anxiety.

€€€

That evening after dinner, Doug rested in the bedroom while I watched TV in the family room. Suddenly he stumbled down the hallway to the front door, violently ill, sweating, dizzy, and weak, begging for help.

"Do something. Call an ambulance. If you don't do it now, I'll drive myself." He pushed the front door open and lurched down two steps into the yard. He zigzagged across the lawn.

I grabbed my cell phone and hurried after him.

"Get me to the hospital. Can't you see I'm sick?" Doug yelled at me for the first time in our thirteen-year marriage.

Shocked and stressed to the point of tears, I tried to locate KU's after hours number in my contacts. "Please give me a minute, I need to find the right number, so I take you to the right ER."

"I said call an ambulance right now. Why won't you help me?"

"I'm trying. They might want you to come to the KU emergency room. I don't want to take you to the wrong hospital."

"Just call an ambulance or I'll get in my van and leave.

"Please! No!"

I continued to struggle with my phone. The more I fumbled around, the more anxious, upset, and louder Doug became. He shouted and staggered around, nearly falling down. I expected to see neighbors come out on their porches. It sounded like we were having a terrible drunken fight.

I was panicked and at the end of my rope. I cannot see well to drive at night, so I called our daughter.

"Jill, please help me get Doug to the nearest ER."

"I'm on my way."

"Wait! Never mind, he's getting in the van. I have to call an ambulance."

"I'll meet you at Centerpoint ER. Call me if they're taking him somewhere else."

I hung up and raced to Doug. "Please... I'm calling right now. Wait! They'll be here any minute."

I called 9-1-1 and Doug took his first ambulance ride. Trembling and clutching the steering wheel until my fingers ached, I followed in my car. Jill met us there. The emergency room personnel provided almost instant relief with anti-nausea medicine.

Doug was soon himself. "Jill, I want you to know how much it means that you came to the ER. I'm so sorry I upset you, Evie. I thought I was dying."

€€€

The next day at Doctor Osgood's office, we explained Doug's terrible reaction and visit to the hospital. The nurses were surprised and apologetic. They gave him anti-nausea medicine, and we crossed our fingers. For the rest of his treatment with Vidaza, the nurses administered anti-nausea meds and things went smoothly.

The Locker Room Angels called often during that first week and boosted Doug's morale. To make him feel even better, Doug's daughter, Katey, came for a visit. She lives in New York and we don't get to see her very often. We picked her up at the airport Thursday night, and she accompanied her dad to his Friday treatment, giving me the day off. When they returned home, Doug had a spring in his step and an ear-to-ear smile. He was free of the port in his forearm. No treatments for three weeks. We were going out to dinner, then to visit the grandkids. Happy Friday.

Running Out of Time?

On Monday, the clinic called to let us know The Worldwide Registry had turned up a couple hundred potential donors. Praise God! The next step was to request funding in order for further tests to be performed on three of the candidates. We were full of hope, but impatient with God's prolonged timing.

When his treatment allowed, Doug continued to work at KC Quality Products, the small industrial brooms and brushes business he owned. He worked hard to keep up with sales calls, deliveries, and everything else it took to keep his customers happy. I could see the stress and fatigue building when he came home from work exhausted.

The Locker Room Angels continued to check in regularly. His best friend on the hockey team, Roy, called often, even though he was spending the winter in Florida. Through the macho nonsense they discussed, I heard care and concern. Doug's mood always improved after those calls.

The last week of February, we got news that funding had been approved for further testing of three young men. All Beth could reveal to us were their ages: one was twenty-six, and the other two were thirty-three. Doug joked that with such young blood, he'd play hockey until he was 100. The waiting wasn't over, but a huge piece of the puzzle dropped into place. We relaxed a bit.

I was overwhelmed with appreciation for these three young men willing to interrupt their busy lives to save the life of a stranger. I prayed one of them would be the one, and we could get "the show on the road," as Doug said.

With that good news came bad. Doug's bloodwork showed his hemoglobin (HGB) was down to 5.8. Typically, HGB under eight was cause for a transfusion. Once again, Doug's stellar fitness and willpower enabled him to function at that low level. Doctor Osgood wanted to hold off on a transfusion as long as possible. The fewer antibodies from transfusions, the better it was for the transplant.

The following week, I emailed Beth for an update. I dreaded 4:30 when Doug would be home from work.

"Hi, have you heard anything?" Doug asked with a smile.

"Beth just responded to my email. No news. She warned me lead time would be weeks, even after the donor is found."

"Oh no!" He dumped his briefcase on the kitchen table, plopped down in his chair, put his elbows on the table and his face in his hands. "I feel like I'm getting worse and worse. I don't know how long I can wait. What if I can't make it til they find someone?"

"Don't say that. You'll make it, honey. She said if she didn't hear anything by the end of the week, she'd find out if we can look at additional donors."

"Well once again, there's nothing I can do but wait and get stuck with needles. The news keeps getting worse, and I'm more and more exhausted."

I shuddered, knowing Doug's condition was declining. Even he admitted that now. Vidaza was not keeping the blasts—quickly dividing cancer cells—at bay.

A late February snowstorm made driving difficult. Doug smiled when he cancelled his blood draw, happy for a chance to delay more bad news. He sat in the family room and picked up a book, content to stay inside the house. That worried me. Normally, he would have cleared off the cars and shoveled the driveway before eight am. Then he'd slip and slide to work and scoop the space in front of his office. He finally ventured out after lunch, and I joined him. Thankfully, the snow was light and fluffy. We enjoyed the lovely winter wonderland.

The next morning, he seemed better. He shoveled the snow that had accumulated overnight and went to his office.

Doug continued to have his blood counts checked often, and his HGB dropped slowly without interruption.

∈∈∈

"Your blood count is really low this morning. I want to check with Doctor Osgood before you leave. Please be seated for a moment." The nurse marched down the hall toward the doctor's office.

"Now what?" Doug said as we looked at each other.

"He wants to see you." The nurse said when she returned. "Please follow me." She settled us in an exam room. In no time, the doctor entered.

"Doug, we need to schedule a transfusion before you get chemo next week. We can't let your counts get any lower."

"But I thought you said transfusions were bad for the transplant."

"That's true. Best-case scenario is not to have lots of transfusions before the procedure. But your count is so low, you need one. You'll feel much better, and I promise it won't hurt your chances for a successful transplant. Hopefully, they'll settle on a donor soon." He moved toward the door. "I'll have my office call the hospital and set up an appointment as soon as possible. My nurse will give you a call." The doctor rushed from his unplanned appointment with us.

"Well, that's a bummer. You have to endure yet another procedure we weren't expecting." I patted Doug's shoulder.

"No kidding, but maybe it won't be too bad. I sure like the idea of feeling better. I'm really struggling through my days lately."

A Dinner Date to Remember

Doug's worsening condition escalated our impatience for an available donor. We needed one now. It was all we could think or talk about. We focused on our gratitude for people around the world who generously donated the gift of hope. The concerns, good wishes, and prayers of family and friends were blessings hidden among the fears and trials of this difficult time. Their love was a treasure we kept uncovering as we went through days of uncertainty. The Locker Room Angels were a huge bright spot for Doug. He called me several times a day to see if I had heard from Beth. The disappointment in his voice each time I said, "No" broke my heart.

On March 1st, the night before the transfusion, Doug and I had a dinner date at Zio's. As we perused the menu, Doug sighed and laid his on the table.

"I feel my chances slipping farther away every day. How long can I keep taking Vidaza? I don't think it's helping. What if they don't find a donor in time?" He reached out to hold my hand across the table.

"Hey now, worrying and thinking the worst are my jobs. Quit trying to horn in."

"I feel so helpless and out of control."

"Me too. This waiting is pure torture." I squeezed his hand.

"It's driving me crazy. I can barely concentrate at work."

"They'll find one, honey. Remember Beth said the odds are excellent."

"Then why is it taking so long?" He withdrew his hand and opened his menu again.

The server approached with a smile and a hello. We returned her greeting. I thought about how normal we appeared despite all that was going on in the background. Oh, how I longed to be that—a normal couple.

After we ordered, I checked the messages on my iPhone. I expected to come up empty as I did countless times a day. Beth's optimism aside, it seemed more likely our miracle would never happen with each passing day. I dropped the phone on the table, gasped, and covered my mouth with both hands. Tears dampened my cheeks.

"What's wrong Evie?"

Speechless, I handed the phone to Doug. His face lit up as he grinned.

"This is huge. It changes everything. I was about to give up. Can you believe it? Two donors are ten out of ten—perfect matches."

It was all we could do not to shout WOO HOO! I pumped my fist. Tears flowed freely. The server ambled over to see if we were okay.

"My husband needs a bone marrow transplant, and we just got word they've found a donor."

"Oh how wonderful! Congratulations!" I noticed her eyes glisten as this stranger shared our triumph. "I'll be back in a minute with your appetizer." She patted my shoulder and wiped her cheek as she turned and walked back to the bar area. After a brief exchange between the waitress and the bartender, he looked over and gave us two thumps up.

"Now we can begin the fight," my man of action said. "Waiting has been killing me— literally."

"I'm so excited. I can barely work up worry about the transfusion tomorrow."

"Really? That's hard to believe. You're so good at it." Doug teased with a bigger grin than I had seen in a long time.

"I can't help it. You have to admit I've had plenty to worry about lately."

"I know. I hate to put you through this. If it helps, I'm not freaked out about tomorrow. Doc said it's no big deal, and I'll feel a lot better. Looks like it'll be the only one I need."

We ordered two glasses of wine and toasted the beginning of the cure.

Finally a Schedule

The transfusion took several hours, but it went well. Doug felt the results the next day. It was amazing to see. He didn't get short of breath walking up the stairs from the basement. We went for a thirty-minute walk with some moderate inclines. He managed it well.

"I feel as if I'm ready to play hockey." Doug said as he breezed through the front door.

"I hate to be a spoil sport, but not today. You'll be busy getting chemo. It'll be interesting to see what your labs say this afternoon. The way you're acting, they'll probably be incredible."

"Let's hope this is the last dose of Vidaza I'll need. I don't know what comes next, but anything will be better than this endless waiting."

"I'll second that."

Doug jumped in the shower and dressed quickly. He found me in the kitchen making lunch. "I'm adding blood donors to the list of people we're grateful for. I feel so much better. The nurse was great, wasn't she? Even the hospital lunch tasted good." Doug left the room to pack his bag with snacks and a book to pass the time during chemo.

I was over the moon to see Doug so close to normal. His mood was better than it had been for weeks. Our home seemed filled with hope.

I checked email for the tenth time that morning. I found a short message from Beth. Some additional donor testing was required to figure out the best match. Knowing little about that side of the process, I prayed at least one of the two donors would schedule those tests soon.

While we were at the Lee's Summit clinic for Doug's infusion, I received an email from the KU clinic about a meeting scheduled for the following day. I looked over at Doug. His closed eyes didn't necessarily mean he was sleeping. I came to recognize it as a sign to keep quiet. He wanted to get through the process his own way.

"Doug is it okay to talk to you about the meeting tomorrow or are you too sleepy?"

"Of course. What meeting?"

"The nurse's email didn't provide a lot of details. I assume at least part of the meeting will be devoted to the timing of the transplant. This will be difficult and long. But I'm so excited for it to begin, so it can end," I said.

"Yeah, I hear you. As they say, 'It'll feel so good when it quits hurtin'. Which reminds me I have to have another bone marrow biopsy, don't I?"

"I think so. After that it could be two to three weeks until the transplant is scheduled." I moved closer to his recliner and patted his leg. "I feel such relief to know this is finally going to happen."

€€€

Doug and I sat in the clinic office waiting for Beth. I thought about the email she had sent the previous day, explaining the next steps. At last, we had a tentative schedule. In four weeks, Doug would have a thorough physical examination, then meet with a psychologist and a social worker. I wished good luck to all three of them. Doug had little patience for talking about this stuff. He wanted to git 'er done.

During those meetings, they explained many of our—mostly my—questions about visitors, isolation, emotions, length of time, whatever we wanted to know. I took a notebook full of questions with me. It took two days to complete this step.

Two or three weeks after that appointment, Doug would enter the hospital for a week's worth of intensive chemo. This chemo would prepare him for the transplant, which had to happen as soon as the chemo was completed. Doug would endure an approximately thirty-day exile in the hospital. I prayed not only for Doug to have patience with his incarceration, but also for the staff. It would take loads of stamina to keep watch on Doug as he plotted his escape.

Beth's voice pulled me from my thoughts. "Good morning," she said as she walked into the room. "Good news. We should know your appointment date this week. They have at least two donors standing by in case the final test finds any problems with the first donor."

"Good," Doug said. "I don't think I can take any more setbacks. I'm ready. Let's do this."

Beth smiled, and promised to get back with us as soon as she learned the date." Oh, by the way, one of the matches being considered is a woman. I'll see you soon."

I snickered. "Oh boy, I'll have to buy you a pink hockey jersey. The locker room will be ruthless if that actually happens."

€€€

Our oldest son, Jason, and his family had recently moved home from California. They now lived about ten minutes from KU hospital. They promised to have my room ready by the time chemo started.

"I'm so happy the kids can offer you a home away from home so close by. I know this isn't easy for you either, but it feels like things are falling into place." Doug put his arm around me as we walked into the elevator.

"From what I understand, timing is crucial. Once the donor is able to confirm a date, everything will be set in motion." I pushed P2 for the parking garage.

"I'm so glad to be done with outpatient chemo. I'm tired of being stuck with that IV needle."

€€€

On March 12th, the waiting was over. We had a plan! On April 2nd and 3rd, Doug would go through pre-transplant testing. He'll get the works. Pulmonary function tests would measure how well his lungs took in and exhaled air, how efficiently they transferred oxygen into his blood. An electrocardiogram would check for problems with his heart's electrical activity. An echocardiogram, which is an ultrasound test, would create images of his heart so the docs could see if everything was normal. He would also have a chest X-ray.

We talked about finances and a social worker did a work-up. Last but not least, another bone marrow biopsy. The doctors would soon know everything there was to know about Doug.

I held Doug in a tight hug. "I expected to be relieved and I am, but I'm also freaked out. How are you taking this so well? You're the one who's going through it."

"What's the point of worrying? I have to do it. I'd be lying if I said I wasn't scared, but mostly I'm glad to finally get started."

"This feels like a real turning point in our lives—as big as finding out about the matching donors, but that felt wonderful. This is scary as hell, and as surreal as when we found out you had leukemia."

"Remember, I'd probably be dead by now if this option wasn't available."

"You sure know how to straighten me up."

On April 15th Doug would sign the consent form. Then everything on our end would be ready for the donor to agree to a date. Doug would be admitted to the hospital shortly after that. He would start his preparation chemo about the same time the donor began the process of donating his or her stem cells.

Doug continued to amaze me with his courage. He was able to cope emotionally and physically. We were both surprised and alarmed when the results from his latest blood test dropped again. He had been full of energy, so we assumed everything was fine. We both expected him to make it to the transplant date without another transfusion. The nurse didn't seem worried. She said he did not need another blood draw until the following week. I put my trepidation on hold. A month from now, Doug would probably be in the hospital. I prayed he would feel good until then and that time would pass quickly.

Doug's mom and sister, Gin, scheduled a visit for the second week of April. Our daughter, Jamie, who lives in Colorado, planned to come later in the month with our two young granddaughters. I always enjoyed visits from family, but I looked forward to those visits with extra excitement.

March 22nd turned out to be a day to remember. We celebrated birthdays for our oldest grandson, Tom, and Kay, but Doug got the best gift. Beth emailed that the donor's physical tests were scheduled for April 8th. If all went well, he could be cleared by the 15th and his cells would be collected on April 25th."

Meanwhile Doug would start medications on April 16th and be admitted to the hospital on April 17th at six am. After all the waiting, turmoil, and anxiety, we were officially on the schedule for his bone marrow transplant.

€€€

Doug and I sat on the couch in the family room a few days later. "Wow! Now that the schedule's set, the days seem to be flying by." He put his arm around me.

"That's a good thing, right?" I snuggled close.

"Sure, but..."

"It's scary isn't it? We'll be regulars at the hospital starting next week. So many tests."

"Yeah and I'll bet most of them involve needles. I'm glad Gin and Mom have plans to visit. That'll distract me. I don't know how much time and energy I can give Jamie and the girls when they come."

"Honey, don't worry about that. They're not coming to be entertained. They want to support us, and I can use it."

"I know, but I doubt I'll be able to be Silly Papa. There's just too much on my mind."

"Doug, everyone understands how serious this is. We know your focus will be to fight through this."

I had other things on my mind as well. One week from today, Doug had a big surprise coming.

Locker Room Angels Make a Plan

Ric, better known as Lutzie, was the organizer of the hockey teams and Bob was second in command. As promised in Lutzie's surprise email, they had met with the teams one night in February 2013. Ric called me to confirm everyone was on board. I choked and wiped tears from my cheeks. "Thank you so much! Any gesture from you guys will mean the world to Doug." Weeks later, after many phone calls and emails, I began to understand the scope of their plan. Remarkably, much of the hockey community in the Kansas City area rallied for a buddy who had a battle on his hands.

I can keep secrets if I have to, but a poker face doesn't come easy. As soon as I buy a Christmas present, I wrap it and put it away so I'm not tempted to give it early.

One day while I was on the phone with Bob, Doug walked into the room. I stopped mid-sentence.

"Is Doug there?"

"Yes." I could feel my face getting hot.

"So do you think you could come in next Wednesday for your hair appointment? Although I like your hair just as it is."

"I'll check and get back to you." I giggled. I felt instant friendship with a man I had never met. Bob ended up being my primary contact. He typed Hair Appointments and Other Stuff in the subject line of his emails. That always made me laugh.

The closest I came to blowing the surprise was right after we bought a Smart TV. Doug was at work, and I was feeling cocky. I grabbed the wireless keyboard and opened my email on the big screen. As I struggled to maneuver the mouse, I heard Doug open the storm door. What was he doing home so early? In seconds, he would be in the family room. There it was—an email from Bob in huge letters. Doug couldn't miss it even without glasses. I jabbed at the keys but could not find the one that got rid of the evidence. Finally, the window closed just as Doug walked within view of the screen.

€€€

Bob regularly updated me on their progress. Each contact made it clearer how generous the plan was. This amazing group of men put together a fundraiser. Players would pay a fee to play two games, plus compete for trophies in a Speed Skating and Hardest Slap-Shot contest. Post-game beer and BBQ would follow. The event also included a raffle.

All proceeds, including a $5 admission fee and any donations would be for a project of my choosing. This event was to be a total surprise to Doug. The goal was to finish the project while Doug was in the hospital recovering from the transplant scheduled for the middle of April. I suggested improvements to the basement, giving Doug a bigger world when he returned home from his month long stay in the hospital. He would be immuno-suppressed and unable to go anywhere or stay alone for at least one hundred days post-transplant.

€€€

The Angels scheduled The Doug Kalvelage Speed Tournament, honoring Doug as the fastest guy on the team, for March 29th at the Independence Event Center in the Missouri Mavericks ice arena. My growing excitement as the day approached made it harder and harder to keep the secret. Doug's arrival at the right moment was my only job, and I didn't want to blow it.

One Saturday, in between errands, I turned to my husband.

"The grandkids have a program at the Independence Events Center on Friday, and they really want us to come. I know you're tired, but we need to make the effort."

"What is it?"

"I don't really know details, just the time and place. I think it has something to do with the school choir." I looked away. Even good lies are difficult.

"Well, I should go since I have no idea what my future holds. It might be a long time before I can attend their activities again."

The lump in my throat felt as if I had swallowed a golf ball. It kept me quiet. He verbalized so little about what he faced. I had to guess what he was thinking. Little comments like this gave me more insight than I wanted.

Doug stared straight ahead at the interstate. "By the way, if this doesn't turn out the way we want it to, please know how much I love you—how glad I am that you're my wife."

Oh great, now was not the time for me to hear a comment like that. I turned to the window, choked back a sob and wiped away tears. I had to get a grip.

During one of Kay's check-in calls, she told me she was coming for the tournament. I let out a huge sigh of relief.

"Oh Kay, that's great for many reasons, but especially because you can help me get him there at the right time and keep me from blowing the surprise. Bring your game face. I'll tell Doug you're coming for a visit. He has no reason to question the timing."

She proved to be a master at keeping Doug busy so we didn't leave the house too early on the big night. I was free to pace and worry while Kay and Doug watched Michigan basketball.

Kay ushered us out the door with perfect timing. After a short drive, we arrived at the arena. I was in the back seat ready to explode with excitement.

"I need to stop at the ladies' room."

"That's no surprise," Doug said. "We'll wait here."

I didn't have to stall long. Shortly after I entered the restroom, the all-clear call buzzed on my phone. I hesitated a moment, then joined Doug and Kay. The three of us trudged up the stairs to the arena. I stood behind Doug to hide my tearful face and pounding heart. Hockey players filled the ice. Grinning family and friends stood and faced Doug.

He stopped dead in the aisle. I stepped next to him, slid my arm through his, and looked up at him. It took a moment. Then Doug's face turned white and he started shaking. His hand covered his mouth. He turned to me. "Is this for me? Is this for me?"

A child handed me a bouquet. I was completely lost in the unfolding scene. About sixty players skated to our end of the rink, banging their sticks on the ice and then against the Plexiglas in a salute to Doug. That did it. I could no longer blink back my tears. I let them flow freely. I'll never forget that moment.

Doug had a wonderful time greeting, hugging and thanking everyone. He kept repeating, "I can't believe anyone went to so much trouble for me. I just don't believe this. Look at all these people." He turned to me. "How in the world did you keep a lid on this?"

The Angels were elated they had pulled off a complete surprise. Pictures of Doug's reaction posted on Facebook left no doubt.

Though he figured out it was a fundraiser, Doug never questioned me about the money. It was easy to keep the rest of the surprise under wraps. Part two was to complete a project of my choosing while Doug was in the hospital.

My husband walked around for days, overwhelmed at what his buddies had done for him. He shook his head in disbelief. Tears of gratitude shone in his eyes at the number of friends and family who had come to this event—for him. What a great mindset to help us through the next three weeks as we waited for Doug to enter the hospital on April 17th.

Final Prep Begins

Jill set us up on a website called CaringBridge. It's a free personal website for patients who face long difficult journeys with health issues. It provides an easy to use journal that allows updates on patient progress, and it has a guestbook—a place where family and friends can leave messages for the patient and caregivers.

I started the journal as soon as we had the schedule. Doug used it to thank everyone who had been a part of the incredible Doug Kalvelage Speed Tournament:

"To all those who participated in and made possible my very special Friday night at the Independence Events Center—thank you, thank you, thank you! I'm still stunned that so many people would go to so much trouble and effort to help create one of the most special events in my life. I wish there was a way to personally thank each and every one of you. You should also know that you made the night very special for someone else—the guy who went to the effort years and years ago to build a small ice rink in the backyard of his house so his kids could learn to skate and play hockey—my dad. He passed away a number of years ago, but I'm sure he's smiling at what he saw on Friday night. Please know he sends his regards. Again, thank you!"

€€€

Doug was still flying high when April 2nd arrived. With butterflies in our stomachs, we drove to KU not knowing what to expect. We went to several departments within the hospital as the doctors gave Doug a thorough going over. For the most part, it was painless.

"Even though it was a long day, that wasn't too bad." Doug said, as we climbed into the van for the drive home.

"Way better than I expected. Nothing they did to you seemed painful or invasive. I feel so much better after talking to the financial person. It sounds like insurance will cover all of this. What a relief!" I sighed.

"Yeah, no kidding. I don't know what tomorrow will be like. I hate to spend all day at the hospital. I'd rather go to the office and get some work done. Actually, I'd rather do a lot of things than go back tomorrow."

"I guess we shouldn't complain. This is what we've been waiting for." I leaned my head back and closed my eyes.

€€€

Tomorrow turned out to be brutal. Doug was in great shape, not a hint of middle age spread. Unlike me, he never overeats, has no concept of why anyone would. However, when he's hungry he doesn't tolerate delays. He had to skip breakfast because of an early morning fasting blood draw, after which he had a physical. Then we rushed off to a class that would educate us on what to expect after the bone marrow transplant. The information provided by the various nurses, social workers, dietitians and other specialists flabbergasted me. They downplayed nothing. We heard the straight story, and it was overwhelming.

As I followed along in a giant binder on the table in front of me, I glanced around. I felt deep sympathy for the young patients and caregivers who, like us, were hearing these details for the first time. How could they possibly care for a young family under these conditions? It was going to be all I could handle to deal with Doug's needs, never mind having children in the house. I prayed they all had family and friends who would share this enormous responsibility.

Everything we heard seemed worse than we had imagined. Doug's restrictions might last much longer than we anticipated, and precautions were impossibly strict. Being a rule person, I planned to adhere to everything completely. However, I would need to study what appeared to be a 10,000 page manual to know what was involved. I couldn't possibly absorb all the recommendations that came at me during the meeting. Help! Where can I get a Cliff Notes version?

Several friends from church offered to bring in meals after Doug's hospital stay was over. I was thrilled to accept their offers. Now I found out that meals brought in from the outside were taboo.

"Protecting the patient from germs is paramount," Beth said. "There's no way you can possibly control the kitchens of other people. No offense meant to well-meaning family and friends, but the consequences are too serious to take chances." She paused and looked at each person seated around the table. "Food gifts must be pre-wrapped or pre-packaged frozen, nothing homemade."

What a disappointment and huge responsibility! Beth nixed one of our favorite pastimes. No eating out for at least 100 days. How could I be sure my kitchen was safe? It was time to stock up on antiseptic wipes.

Beth continued, "It's necessary to keep all food surfaces: stove, dining table, dishpans, and counter tops squeaky clean. The same for bathroom areas. If practical, it's best that the patient have his own bathroom."

She urged us to remove all plants, pets, and rugs from the areas where Doug spent most of his time. If possible, all pets—especially cats and birds needed to be adopted out for the infamous 100 days. It was best to put knick-knacks and other nonessential items away so I could easily keep the house clean. Linens required frequent washing. Maintenance of Doug's minivan was essential to avoid dust, pollen and other irritants. Home and vehicle windows had to remain closed and time outside kept to a minimum. Was this really possible?

A huge sigh escaped from Doug. I scribbled a note to him. "This is crazy. I don't know how we can possibly do it."

He shrugged his shoulders and wrote back. "No big deal."

Clearly, he wasn't taking any of this to heart. Hadn't he been listening? Getting my husband to adhere to these rules was going to be the challenge of my lifetime, and I had raised four kids. I knew any time he felt good, he would sneak into his normal zone, scorning any precautions that didn't make sense to him.

What did that social worker say? We needed to live within thirty minutes of the hospital or stay at a special lodge provided for patients who lived farther away. Hmm. While it would be nice to stay at home, I secretly hoped our house was too far away. I would have immediate help if something went wrong.

Suddenly, Doug stood up and announced, "I'm done with this meeting. I'm hungry and I'm going to get lunch right now." He marched toward the door. No one challenged him. They just stared.

I waved to Doug. "I'll meet you downstairs when the meeting is over." I looked around the table. "Sorry," I sheepishly apologized to the group and the meeting continued.

After the nurse dismissed us, I found Doug in the cafeteria eating a hamburger and fries. "That was quite a dramatic exit."

"Did I miss much? I was just so hungry and that crap was getting to me. We have plenty of time to learn about how long and miserable this is going to be. Enough is enough for one day."

"No, you didn't miss much. You're right. They can't expect us to learn all this in one day. We have thirty days to ask questions. We'll know the drill by the time you leave the hospital. By the way, how far are we from KU?"

"About twenty-five minutes. Why?"

"Did you hear them mention that if we live more than thirty minutes from the hospital, we're supposed to stay at the Hope Lodge?"

"Oh for Pete's sake, don't be silly. We live plenty close enough. Why would you want to stay there instead of in our own home?"

"Again, you're the voice of reason. I'm just so nervous about taking care of you. They've scared me half to death with all the precautions today."

"Ple-e-eze don't worry. We'll do fine. We aren't the first people to have to do this or the dumbest."

"We're so blessed to live in a time when this is possible. I'm eternally grateful to the young man who is donating. Without this treatment, I could have lost you by now."

"Well you didn't. Let's not think about that."

Doug was right. My mind was already on the edge without borrowing trouble. My early morning devotions developed into a must. That time of reading, prayer, and journaling each day kept me in touch with my gratitude. I came to see thankfulness as the antidote to worry and depression. I understood that without God, a loving family and friends, and the wonderful staff at KU, it wouldn't be possible for me to survive. The worry and stress were beyond my capacity, but prayers, smiles, and support in the form of calls, emails, and guest book entries in CaringBridge kept me believing we would get through this terrible ordeal.

Best Laid Plans

A few days after the tournament and all the hospital appointments, I drove to Pittsburgh, Kansas about two hours from Kansas City, to attend the three-day Christian Writers Fellowship (CWF) conference. I met Linda, my writing sidekick, who had driven in from Tulsa.

That evening, I talked to Doug. He was still reveling in the fact that his buddies had pulled off such an awesome event.

The next morning during a break, I noticed I had missed a call from Doug. I slipped into the hallway and dialed his cell.

"Hi, Hon, it's me. Great conference. Linda and I are really enjoying it. I missed your call. Is everything okay?"

Silence.

"Hello Doug, are you there? Are you okay?" Panic seized me. I drew in a sharp breath.

"No."

"No? Oh my gosh! What's wrong?"

"The doctor called about thirty minutes ago. They got the biopsy results. Evie, I have Stage Four Leukemia. He told me to get to the KU Hospital right away, bypass admissions, and come directly to the fourth floor. They'll meet me in Room 4206."

"Oh no! You can't drive yourself. You need someone with you. I can't believe this happened when I'm not there." I slid down the wall and landed on the floor.

"It's okay. I called Roy. I'm packing. He'll be here in a few minutes. I don't know what to throw in my duffel bag. Don't know how long I'll be there. Don't know anything, except that it can't be good when a doctor calls you personally and tells you to get to the hospital now."

"Thank God Roy can take you. I'll be there as soon as I possibly can. I wish I hadn't come to the conference." I hung up and stared into space.

"There you are. I wondered where you wandered off to... Oh Evie, what's wrong?" Linda grabbed my shoulders.

My heart raced, and I couldn't stop trembling. "I have to leave now. Doug's on his way to the hospital. His leukemia has gotten worse."

"Oh no, what can I do? Should I drive you?" She pulled me to my feet and walked me toward the lobby. "How would we get your car back home?"

"No. I have to do this. Help me pack and load my car so I can get out of here."

We stuffed things into my suitcase and threw everything into the car. She sent me on my way with a hug, a prayer, and a command to drive safely.

Once on the road, I cried so hard, I could barely see. I was more afraid and alone than I had ever been. I wished Linda could have come with me.

What did this mean? Was he dying? I pounded the steering wheel until my fist ached and raged at our bad luck. The doctor's words during our initial visit haunted me. "You're in Stage Two, the perfect time for a bone marrow transplant. Stage One is too early for the risk involved. Stages Three and Four make it much more complicated."

Now he was in Stage Four. Things were much more complicated. What did that mean?

I pictured him in a hospital bed, pale, weak, surrounded by nurses and life-saving machines.

My mind was numbed by the reality of a two-hour drive ahead of me with no other choice but to drive it. Thankfully, autopilot kicked into gear. I didn't know the best way to get to the hospital or where in that huge complex to go. We had visited briefly the first time Kay was in town, but Doug always did the driving. I never paid attention. I thought I had plenty of time to learn.

I called my son-in-law, Matt, for directions so I didn't waste time getting lost. He could barely understand me through my sobs, but our conversation helped clear my head. I was able to comprehend the best way to get there. I settled in and drove, exhausted from crying and worry, but focused on what I had to do.

My cell phone rang. It was Roy, calling from the hospital.

"This isn't good. The doctor's made it clear this is very serious. You can't freak out in front of Doug. Valet park in front of the hospital. That'll be easiest."

"Okay. Thanks for being with him, Roy. I'm almost there. See you soon."

I pulled up to the hospital, flustered by multiple lanes and busy traffic. Where in this confusion was valet parking? What should I take in with me? How long would I be here? I parked at the main entrance and got out. A parking attendant walked up to me and put his arm around me.

"Here's your ticket, I'll take care of your car." His kindness started my tears again.

"My ... my husband just arrived here and I... I don't know what to do."

"I could tell by the look on your face. Don't you worry. This is a great hospital. He'll be okay."

Instead of trying to figure out what to take with me, I grabbed everything. Dragging my overnight bag, purse, pillow, and computer bag, I rushed to the automatic doors, nearly crashing into them. I scurried to the elevator, trying not to bang into anyone with my baggage. Up to the fourth floor.

I hustled out the elevator door and down the hall to the bone marrow transplant unit we had visited briefly weeks ago. I hurried through the outer door into the air-locked vestibule and waited for it to close as the sign directed. Then pushed through the inner door, into the hallway like a crazed overloaded bellhop.

Into the bone marrow transplant unit we had visited briefly weeks ago.

"What are you doing?" A nurse rushed out from behind the counter. She stared at me with furrowed eyebrows.

"My husband was just admitted. I have to see him right away."

47

"What's his name?"

I told her. She said he wasn't there. Stupid with anxiety, I stood there immobilized, clueless about what to do next.

"Let me check." The RN stepped behind the workstation and looked him up. "He's in Unit 42, across the hall."

"Sorry." I hustled out.

(Later I would become familiar with the protocol of BMT Unit 41. It was a fluke I was able to burst in like that. The inner door is locked, and the nurse on duty must buzz visitors in after they have completed the proper cleaning protocol. The space between the two doors has a sign-in sheet and a wash station with antibacterial wipes for cleaning purses and other belongings. This protocol is vital to the airlock system, which provides protection against germs for the immunocompromised bone marrow transplant patients.)

Mortified, I hauled my baggage into Unit 42 and dropped it. I saw Roy in the hallway. My daughter-in-law, Becky, rushed to give me a hug.

"Oh Becky, thanks for coming." I held her tight.

"Of course. Call anytime you need me."

Roy led us to a family waiting area. Usually cool and calm, he looked pretty shook-up. That unnerved me even more.

"I need to talk to you before you see Doug," Roy said. "You look horrible. Calm down. You have to get it together before you see him. He's doing fine, but the doctors didn't have any good news. You're not going to wanna hear what you gotta hear."

Becky gave me another a hug, and tears started again. Roy looked at me and shook his head. "Get your game face on."

We shuffled down the hall toward Room 4206. Nurses smiled, but it was impossible for me to smile back. Pale, exhausted patients pushing walkers stumbled down the hall, dragging IV poles.

A big sign on Doug's door instructed us to clean our hands before we entered. We complied. I knocked gently on the door in case he was sleeping. I nudged the door open and poked my head into the room.

"What the...?" I threw the door open. "I expected you to be flat on your back in bed."

"I'm doing step-ups. I brought my stool, so I could keep up with my exercise as much as possible."

"You're working out like a madman. I thought you were half-dead."

"You sound disappointed." Doug winked.

"I don't know what I am. Of course I'm thrilled you seem to feel good, but sit down and tell me what's happening." I whacked him lightly on the shoulder, then hugged him.

Becky and Roy said good-bye and retreated.

"The doctors are all gloom and doom, but as you can see, I feel fine. A whole team of them just left. I have Stage Four Leukemia." Doug sat on the bed.

"Stage Four? How did that happen so fast?"

Doug's shoulders drooped. "It just happened."

"Remember when Dr. Ganguly said you were in the perfect stage for a transplant. Stage Three and Four made it riskier, and Stage One wasn't bad enough?

"Sometimes I wish you didn't have such a good memory."

"Can you even have the transplant?" I leaned forward in my chair and held his hands.

"I can't have it in three weeks like we planned, but I can still have it."

"Thank God."

"I gotta have chemo first to kill the cancer cells. I'll be here at least two weeks, most likely a month. They want me to be part of a clinical trial. What do you think?"

"Two weeks? A month? Then what? What's the clinical trial for?" I closed my eyes and combed both hands through my hair.

"Just settle down please." He patted my knee. "They want to evaluate different combinations and intensities of chemotherapy. I don't know exactly what's it all about. I don't get to choose. It's a blind trial. If it works, they'll reschedule the transplant for May."

"If …?"

"They're pretty sure they can get this under control, but it complicates things and won't be fun. What do you think about the trial?"

"Don't we have enough to deal with? I haven't even fully processed the fact you've gotten worse. The plan we waited months for is down the drain. Now they want to add a new twist. My head's spinning. I'm sick about all this." I shrugged my shoulders. "It's up to you." What do you wanna do?" I shook my head to clear it, but there was no way to take it all in. April 17th was not going to happen.

"I think I should do it." Doug lay back against the pillow. "It's a way of giving back."

"Everything was all set and now this." I crossed my arms and bowed my head. "Do you have to decide right now?"

"Pretty much, the doctors need to know before they begin treatment. My decision will affect the chemicals and dosages. They want to start ASAP. The cancer cells are on a rampage."

"I admire your decision. It's the right thing to do." I scooted my chair closer, laid my head on his chest, and prayed.

The Roller Coaster Begins

Doug handled the news better than I expected—two months in the hospital instead of one. He signed the consent form for the clinical trial, and chemo was set to begin soon. My husband settled into this small world—a tiny room with two windows that looked onto a black roof a few feet below. Even birds refused to fly into that dismal view. No trees. No grass. No cars. No people walking about. An uncomfortable hospital bed, tray table, recliner, and a couch that opened into a hard, cramped sleeping surface filled his space. The distressing accommodations also included a closet and a bathroom. The latter was off limits to anyone except the patient. Once chemo started, Doug would be highly susceptible to germs. My powder room lived outside Unit 42 and down a long hallway. I memorized the route and could make the trek with my eyes closed in the middle of the night. I shared it with all the other women visitors to the fourth floor.

€€€

The day after Doug arrived in Unit 42, a team of nurses came into the room. "Since you're left-handed, we're going to place a peripherally-inserted central catheter (PICC) in your right arm. This is a sterile procedure only physicians or other specially trained medical personnel perform." The team wore gowns, masks, and gloves.

I heard the word sterile. "Should I leave the room?" I asked.

"No, that's not necessary. We do need you to put on a mask and move to the opposite side of the room."

That was fine with me. I had no stomach for watching the procedure.

The nurse handed both of us masks. "Doug, you need to put one on as well."

The nurse put on her own mask and turned to Doug. "We'll advance a line through your vein until the tip rests above your heart in the superior vena cava a large vein that goes to your heart."

Doug nodded.

My knees buckled, and I leaned against the wall.

"PICCs can be left in place much longer than regular IV's, which are shorter and remain in place only for a few days. We'll be able to use this line for long-term treatment of pain, infection, nutrition, blood draws, or chemotherapy. It'll have three ports so you won't have to be stuck so often."

"Yay. Now you're talking. I'm all for that." Doug turned his head and smiled at me.

"This PICC will be in place for months. Any questions?"

That's always my cue. "Will this replace that horrible thing that sticks out of patients' chests? My brother and my best friend had something like that."

"Yes. We'll use the PICC instead. What they had is a tunneled catheter. In that case, we surgically insert one end into a vein in the neck or chest with the other end outside the skin."

I shuddered. God must have known I couldn't handle one of those. I'll be forever grateful Doug's was in his arm. I get squeamish looking at simple IV's, much less something that sticks out of a neck or chest. Considering the other options—constant sticks or a tunneled catheter— I forced myself to get used to the PICC in his arm. Doug adjusted to it right from the beginning. Apparently, anything was better than all the needles he had dealt with up until now.

Since his PICC covered chemotherapy, hydration, and other needed fluids, an IV pole was his constant irritating companion. He dubbed it IVY. She accompanied him on his walks in the hall and even to the bathroom. That first day, we got a taste of the hospital nightlife we would experience during the coming weeks. Hydration was an important part of the plan. Bathroom trips all night escalated our sleep interruptions beyond the normal hospital routines—blood draws and vital sign monitoring.

The PICC was a blessing, but sometimes all three ports were in use or a certain blood test required a fresh stick. As a result, Doug still endured many needles.

"I need to draw blood, and I can't use the PICC for this." The nurse said glumly. "Oh my, you have garden hose veins. This'll be super easy." Her face brightened.

Doug and I looked at each other and rolled our eyes. "We've heard that before," my husband whispered.

Though the nurses drooled at the sight of his large veins, his garden hoses were full of valves that blocked the needle. In addition, unless held firmly in place, his veins rolled, escaping the poke. We learned that some nurses and phlebotomists—medical workers trained in drawing blood from a vein—are needle wizards while some are not.

"Don't count. Don't tell me when you're gonna do it. Just do it! Get it right the first time." Those words became Doug's hostile mantra every time he had to be stuck. Even some of the veteran nurses gave up after several attempts. Following frustrated protests in which Doug blew up several times, the IV team took over. Whenever Doug required phlebotomy, the staff called them. Things were tense enough without Doug enduring multiple sticks.

€€€

I watched my husband as he paced his room, did squats and step-ups, then plopped on the bed.

"This is a prison cell, and I've done nothing wrong."

"I wish I had good news, honey. I talked to the nurse. Still no beds available in a bigger room. You were a bit of an emergency. It wasn't like they could wait until a better room opened up."

"I know, but they can't expect me to live here for thirty days. I can't even go to the unit family room for a change of scenery."

"That garbage dump? Yuck! I can't believe how people leave their chaos for someone else to deal with. There's always trash around, the counters and tables are sticky and full of crumbs. Coffee, soda, and water splotches accumulate on the floor waiting for housekeeping. That's the last place I'd want you to be." I sat next to him and gave him a side hug.

"The days are dragging, and it's only the beginning. All the rules! No grandkids under twelve. What's that all about?"

"The nurse explained kids are germ factories. Remember? I can't imagine how tough this is for you. Believe me having so many restrictions is hard on me too. I'd love some company. No one wants to chance a visit and make you sick."

"I hate that you're isolated from your girlfriends and family because of me."

"Don't worry about me. I'm fine. You have enough on your plate." I kissed his forehead. "By the way, the door to one of the corner rooms was open when I came in this morning. I peeked in. It had patient belongings inside, so it wasn't available. The occupant must have been out of the unit for tests or something. The point is, it looked huge and had lots of big windows—a much better room as we suspected."

Doug straightened up. "Really? Oh, man! Wouldn't that be great? I'll remind the nurse I'm interested in a transfer ASAP." He slumped again. "Every time I ask if there's a corner room available they say there isn't. At least they let me walk the hall around the nurses' stations."

And he did. Lap after lap after lap.

I noticed patients walking the big hall outside the unit, even taking the elevator down to get some fresh air outside the hospital. Why couldn't Doug? It wasn't fair. Were our doctors too rigid? I didn't dare mention it to Doug until I checked with someone.

On my next trip to the restroom, I caught a nurse in the hall and quizzed her.

"Doug's receiving chemo to get his leukemia in remission so he can have the transplant. His immune system will drop very low." The nurse explained. "Other patients in this unit aren't in his situation. This unit houses patients with a variety of needs. A few like Doug are getting ready for a transplant. Others will complete their treatment here and some will breathe their last breath here. I know it's hard for him to be so isolated, but it's just not worth the risk."

"I didn't realize that." I hung my head. Now I understood why I saw small children in the halls. They were here to say good-bye to loved ones. I wiped away a tear, regretting my uninformed judgements.

I told Doug what the nurse said. We both assumed there would be a turnover for good or bad reasons, but the unit remained full.

We limited our hall exercise to times when no children were around. On our walks, we looked longingly at the large corner rooms. The nurses cheered Doug on as he did his laps, remarking they had never before cared for a patient who didn't have to be encouraged to walk.

After his circuits, Doug read and watched a little TV—when he wasn't doing step-ups or squeezing his handgrips. He called the office daily to check on his assistant, Jean, who was doing an incredible job keeping KC Quality Products, Inc. humming along. With few exceptions, she was able to handle everything. When she had a question, she would call my phone to make sure Doug wasn't napping. He was glad to be part of things when she needed his help.

ϵϵϵ

One day after Doug finished his breakfast and completed his first session of walking the halls, he decided to take a rare nap.

"This bed is so noisy and moves all the time. I can't sleep on it. I guarantee if purchasing agents spent one night on these beds, they'd change out the whole lot of them."

"Honey, the constant movement keeps patients from getting bedsores."

Doug scowled at me and moved over to the couch.

"Good luck." Having spent time trying to sleep on the couch, I could verify it was noiseless, but the cushions were paper-thin. I was unable to keep the sheets tucked. As I tossed and turned, the bedding rolled up into a ball, completely ineffective at keeping me covered and warm.

Later in the day, a nurse showed us how to put the bed into sleep mode. Doug continued to boycott the hospital bed during the day unless he was feeling terrible. Often at night, he asked me to trade with him.

In the darkness, I lived in fear of getting blood drawn or medications I didn't need. Often a nurse would wake me in the night.

"You're not Doug, are you?"

"No, he's over on the couch. Don't think he's being chivalrous giving me the bed. This thing is dreadful."

Caution and Isolation

The nurses' continual reminders played video loops in my overwhelmed mind. "Only two visitors at a time. Be sure to explain to family and friends how susceptible Doug is to germs. Anyone who visits must have no signs of illness. They can be dangerous for Doug even if they've been near someone who is ill. Children under twelve cannot visit. Studies show they're germ factories."

For many weeks, Doug could see only three of our ten grandchildren. He didn't have the patience for Smartphones or Facetime. He liked his flip phone and repeatedly refused my offers to upgrade him for his birthday or Christmas. Even in these isolated circumstances, he remained stubborn. I tried to convince him how fun it would be to see the kids on Facetime. A smartphone would give him an easy way to read the news, watch movies, and research questions. Jill loaned us her brand new IPad to use while he was in the hospital. I enjoyed her generous loan, but drawings and phone calls would have to do for Doug. Stunning artwork from grandchildren ages four through nine plastered the walls of Room 4206. Each masterpiece signed with loads of love to Papa.

Everyone who entered the room: nurses, doctors, housekeepers, and aides—smiled and commented our room boasted the best artwork on the whole floor, possibly the entire hospital. The love represented in those colorful pictures immeasurably cheered us.

Doug felt his confinement more every day. Anxious to exercise, he continued to wear a path in the floor around the nurses' station. The staff smiled at his discipline and ambition.

"Great job. Hope you inspire the other patients."

On my trips down the hall to the large restroom, which served the entire fourth floor, I cringed whenever I noticed a woman leave without washing her hands. Ever vigilant, I feared she might be visiting Doug's unit. My hands were raw from all my handwashing. How dare she be lax in her hygiene?

The messes in the family room upset me more and more. I felt a disturbing amount of anger, and I had to bite my tongue to avoid confronting the rule breakers. I worried I'd lose control of my emotions, which were dangerously frayed. My heart broke to see small kids walk the halls even though I now understood the reason. I finally cornered a nurse and voiced my concerns.

She put her arm around my shoulders. "We do our best to stress handwashing, and cleaning up the family room after each use. I'm sure you've noticed the signs all around."

I huffed an exaggerated sigh. "Yes, I have. I just don't understand people blatantly ignoring them."

"We simply cannot monitor everyone or demand they strictly adhere to the rules. Try not to worry." She patted my back. "Do your best, especially while you're in Doug's room. Remind him to be aware of who's in the hall when he goes for a walk. He'll be fine." She walked away, and then turned back. "In BMT Unit 4109, there will be stricter rules to keep him safe. That's when it really counts."

Doug's neutropenic diet required stringent protocols. He had to avoid bacteria that can be present in food not properly washed and/or stored. Even fresh fruits and vegetables from the cafeteria required proper cleaning. I felt silly washing bananas. Doug couldn't consume outside food or drink unless it was safely packaged. No fountain drinks, Five Guy's burgers or homemade cookies. That restriction would be in force until his blood counts sufficiently recovered after chemo.

"Doug, I'm washing your bananas for Pete's sake. Please don't pick up anything off the floor. The nurse warned you about that yesterday. Ple-e-ez don't put your shoes up on the bed or recliner."

He smiled. "You're a real nag."

I wasn't amused. "Every directive from the nurses and doctors is important in my opinion. You wanna pick and choose the ones that make sense to you?" I threw up my hands in dismay.

Thankfully, most nurses were sensitive to Doug's personality and the frustration he felt at having his independence hijacked. They went out of their way to help Doug feel a part of his treatment, allowing him to make his own decisions when possible. He never wore a hospital gown. When he showered, he split the bottom of a gallon plastic bag, slipped his hand in and secured it with rubber bands instead of wrapping it with Saran Wrap—the typical way to protect a PICC. Doug hates to accept conventional ways of doing things. He always searches for the best tool for the job.

A nurse came in to check on Doug. She must have noticed he was not his cheery self. She sat down to visit.

"This process causes random exhaustion, nausea, chills, fevers, lack of appetite, rashes, and underlying fatigue." She leaned toward Doug. Her eyes glistened with empathy. "All nurses agree cancer treatment is barbaric, but it's all we've got. We look forward to the day when we can provide more humane treatment for our patients. That's why we're grateful for patients like you who agree to clinical trials."

"I figure it's the least I can do to help other people who have to go through this."

€€€

Compassion and encouragement from the medical staff were our lifelines to sanity and hope. They became friends, confidants, cheerleaders, and primary visitors. Family stayed away to avoid contaminating Doug.

Daily ups and downs were frequent and random—just as the nurses promised. Some mornings, he felt great and ate heartily. But by afternoon, he would be exhausted and couldn't eat a bite. He circled through chills, fevers, rashes, and fatigue. As Doug's blood values continued to tank and compromise his immune system, Doug became even more wary of visitors. I respected his feelings and didn't encourage anyone to come. I felt lonely and reclusive.

One Monday morning, a nurse dropped in to bring fresh water and give Doug his meds. "We'll be checking your progress with a bone marrow biopsy in the next few days."

"Yay! I'll finally get a change of scenery. Or do they come to my room?"

"You'll have to go downstairs to radiology, but you'll be lying on a gurney."

"I don't care. At least I'll be on the other side of those doors."

I laughed. "Talk about desperate."

€€€

Doug's next dose of chemo took the wind out of his sails. I touched his shoulder to awaken him for lunch. His eyes flickered open. "Are you feeling okay?" I asked.

"I feel pretty flat, but I'm glad I don't feel sick to my stomach like the nurse said I might."

"Glad to hear you're not nauseated. The spaghetti looks delicious and smells good too. Can you sit up and try some?"

"It does smell pretty good, but I don't have much of an appetite. Why don't you eat it?"

"I hate to do that in case you feel hungry later."

"Order a tray for yourself next time. Go ahead and eat what you want. I ordered a bunch of stuff. Besides the nurses bring me snacks any time I want."

I didn't want to bother him with it, but guest trays were expensive when you considered how many meals I might eat in two months. Eating his extras or grabbing something at the snack bar was cheaper. It was three dollars a day to park. It was silly to worry about the small stuff when we had so much going on, but my parents raised me to be frugal—a hard habit to break.

A New Kitchen

During my next trip home, I scheduled a meeting with the three Angels who were knowledgeable about construction. They came to the house. I was delighted to meet them. We stood in a circle in the kitchen to discuss possibilities.

"My plan is to remodel the basement. I want to make that space comfortable, clean, and safe for Doug. After the transplant, he won't be able to go anywhere for one hundred days."

Bob flinched. "One hundred days. That's brutal."

"That's going to drive Dougie nuts," Bill said.

What is it with grown men, tough hockey players calling each other Bobby, Dougie, Tommy, Timmy, and Lutzie? I guess it fits right in with those pats on the behind, and whatever makes it okay for them to hug each other like European men after they score.

"I can't imagine how antsy he's going to get. That's why I thought a finished basement would double the size of his world and give him a private space away from me—his Man Cave."

"Makes sense." Tim said. "Let's go downstairs and figure out what we can do."

On the way down the stairs, I laid out my plan. "I'd like the floor tiled, the ceiling dropped, new lights installed in dark spots and on the wall next to the steps." I looked at them one by one, as we gathered in the basement. "That's probably twice as much as you raised, but if there's money left over, I have plenty of other ideas. I don't want to be greedy. What do you think? How much would that cost? I have no idea what my budget is or how much stuff costs."

"Whoa!" Bob smiled and put his arm around my shoulders. "Take a breath."

"Okay. Your generosity kicked my imagination and excitement into overdrive."

Bob looked toward Tim. "What do you think?"

"Actually, this basement is nice." The others nodded. "The floor has a few cracks. If you tile it, you run the risk of keeping moisture trapped under it, which will cause more cracking and lift the flooring. It might be better just to clean it really well. The lighting isn't a bad idea."

I hoped my attempt at a smile hid my disappointment. He didn't like my plans. At least that's what I got out of what he said. I didn't know what else to suggest.

"Let's go upstairs," Bob said.

They were charming as we sat around the kitchen table. We talked about Doug, life, kids and spouses. I would never tell them, but it was as comfortable and enjoyable as if they were my girlfriends.

Somehow, my original plan morphed into a kitchen remodel. I was speechless for a moment. Then I argued, "That would be for me. The kitchen's fine as far as Doug's concerned."

"We're all married and we know if Mama's happy—everybody's happy. Besides a new kitchen would do more to increase the property value of your home. Any man can appreciate that."

I pressed my hands on the table and leaned forward. "You don't have to ask me twice. I've wanted a kitchen update for years. Check out this floor." I pointed to the two-toned linoleum. "Doug started to tear out the floor when the fridge leaked. Then he didn't feel well enough to finish it. Since then, we've been a little crazy. I don't know how to thank you guys."

"I'll have Lutzie give you a call with the names of some guys who do this kind of work. You need to get busy picking out what you want for the counter-tops, back-splash and flooring. Do you want to change the cabinets?" Tim asked.

"Sounds great, but this is all so new, I'm stunned. I need time to think."

"We need to give the contractors some lead time. This is a busy time of year. When can we schedule this?"

"I have no idea. The transplant was to be on April 17th but Doug's leukemia got worse. That's why he's in the hospital. It's Stage Four now. They have to give him chemo to get him in remission before they can reschedule."

"Roy sent out an email about that. Darn! What a bummer!" Bill said.

"I don't know what to expect right now. Everything is so up in the air."

"Let me know as soon as you figure out a date," Bob said.

They left and I sat in my recliner. What just happened? A new kitchen? Was that possible? I could see it in my mind's eye. A granite counter-top, new cabinets with lights beneath, a new floor, new blinds. Would Doug like the idea?

€€€

On hurried trips away from the hospital, I shopped for sinks, counter-top material, subway tile, flooring, and paint colors. I met with cabinet people, flooring installers, and painters. My vision came together as evidenced by the photos in my iPhone. My daughter-in-law and I shopped at a granite showroom that felt like an art museum. So many beautiful slabs to choose from. I finally settled on one. Maybe I could afford new appliances to boot. Every time I tried to ask about my budget, Bob cut me off. He said he'd worry about that.

Changes in Doug's treatment plan continued to make it impossible to schedule the work. Until we knew a firm date for his bone marrow transplant, there was no way to begin the remodel. I couldn't be certain how long my kitchen transformation would take.

It seemed reasonable to expect delays in the target date. I had heard many stories that described nightmarish tales of going way past the anticipated completion date. We would be on a strict deadline. Doug could not come home to dust, mold, and other construction contaminants.

Worrying about Doug filled my mind. No brain space to think about my dream kitchen anyway. I felt too stressed to meet with any more contractors. Color and material choices overwhelmed me. I accepted it would be impossible to schedule such a big project until Doug was well. Disappointed yet relieved, I put the project on permanent hold.

Finally—Visitors

A few weeks into our stay, Gin called to say she was going to bring Roz, Doug's mom, to visit. I was over the moon at the thought of visitors.

"Hey Doug! Your mom and Gin will be here tomorrow. Becky's picking them up at the airport."

"I didn't realize it was tomorrow. I'm really looking forward to their visit."

"Time flies when you're having fun."

He gave me a dirty look.

I suffered a little irrational irritation that he was open to them spending time with him, yet he panicked at the thought of local family and friends dropping by. Then again, neither one of them was around a child under twelve. My annoyance didn't last long. I eagerly anticipated their companionship. Besides, Doug was entitled to feel comfortable with whomever.

"We can watch the Michigan game tonight if you can stay awake. Try to get some rest. You may not feel like eating, but at least have a drink of your protein shake."

He took several sips and closed his eyes.

As Doug napped, I pondered what our visitors would say about his appearance. I thought he looked good, even though the hospital routine and medications had drained him. He hadn't lost his hair yet, but the nurses assured us he would soon.

The next morning brought big changes. Doug was exhausted and made only a feeble effort to eat if I coaxed him. He didn't even have the energy to talk to his assistant, Jean, on the phone. For some reason, he refused to nap. He felt chilled. Though the nurses warned us these were possible effects from the chemo, I was alarmed at his lethargy, even compared to yesterday.

That afternoon, just as his mom and Gin arrived, Doug perked up.

"Hmm, I guess you're getting tired of my company. Visitors show up, and you're totally revived."

We visited for several hours and enjoyed the treats Gin brought, all properly packaged. I noticed Doug's eighty-six year-old mom had fallen asleep on the recliner. We talked quietly to allow her a short nap. Doug dosed off and on.

"Gin, did you say you wanted to stay with Doug tonight?" I asked

"I do."

Doug brightened at the news. "That'll give us a chance to catch up. Evie, you'll be able to sleep in your own bed."

"Okay. I'll take your mom to dinner and then home so she can recover from traveling."

€€€

Roz and I had an early dinner at Olive Garden, then drove home for a much-needed good night's sleep. I almost cried when I climbed into my own bed with my comfy pillow. I always appreciated the rare nights at home, but this was different. With Gin on duty, I was worry-free.

I woke up refreshed, and Roz looked better too. We had coffee, a quick breakfast, and prepared for our day at the hospital. For those fifteen hours, life felt normal. But by the time I pulled into the parking structure, my stomach was in knots. How had the night gone? Was he able to eat? Gin didn't call so I'll think the best.

Gin met us at the door of Doug's room. She put her finger to her lips and whispered. "He's sleeping. Let's go into the hall to talk."

Roz took her spot on the recliner as Gin and I stepped out into the hall.

"I understand why you're worried. He's having a hard time eating. They offer him a nice variety any time of the day or night, but he's not interested."

"The nurses are great, aren't they? You can tell working with cancer patients is their passion. I don't know what I'd do without them. Nobody visits, everyone is afraid to make Doug sick."

"It must be hard going through this mostly on your own." Gin hugged me. "Remember Doug's a fighter, and he's in such great shape except for the leukemia. That sounds weird, doesn't it? Maybe he'll force himself to eat."

"That's all true, but it's hard to see him so weak and lethargic."

"No kidding. He's always been such a maniac. I'm stunned to see him so fatigued, but chemo is rough stuff."

"Your being here has been a serious break for me. Doug loves spending time with you. I don't look forward to you leaving in two days."

"Oh, I forgot to tell you. The nurse told us the doctor ordered a different sleeping pill for tonight. They think maybe it's too strong, and that's part of his sleepiness."

"Great! I hope that makes a difference. Thanks again for coming, Gin. I feel like you hit my reset button, and I can begin again."

"I'm glad we came. I wanted to see for myself how you two were doing. Mom needed to see him even though traveling is getting to be too difficult for her." We glanced at her dozing in the recliner.

The next morning, my husband looked remarkably well. He received his last dose of chemo. I couldn't help but think about the fact his original transplant date was less than a week away. I didn't mention it to him, but I imagine he remembered it too. We spent the day watching movies and visiting with his mom and sister.

"I feel better. It had to be the sleeping pill. I even feel like eating."

Gin grinned. "The good news doesn't stop there. They're going to remove the IV pole or as you call it, IVY the rattletrap. I'm relieved things are going well. It makes it a lot easier to leave tomorrow."

My smile faded as I thought about how lonely we would be.

The next day, we said our good-byes and returned to life without visits. Fortunately, Doug retained his appetite, good mood, and energy. Without IVY, he walked the halls as a free man. What a change from a couple days ago! For the time being, the roller coaster cruised on a level plane. I completed an assignment that was due for work. Then I took advantage of Doug's well-being to work on some medical paperwork. We dealt with advanced directives, Power of Attorney, and applications for available programs to help with expenses. I called for a social worker, and he assisted us through that maze.

The next morning, instead of my recent begging prayers, my prayers were full of gratitude for how well Doug seemed. He was reading, and I was writing an optimistic CaringBridge entry when our favorite cheerleader nurse popped into the room.

"Doug, you're a superstar! You're doing so well. But I need to warn you next week you might feel flu-like symptoms, and you'll probably begin to lose your hair. Actually, I hesitate to predict anything about you, the way you continue to reset the bar. I don't ever remember a patient like you. Your exercise, general health, and good attitude make you a unique case." She shook her head and smiled.

"That's why you love me, right?"

"Right."

"Does anyone ever escape without losing their hair?" Doug sat up straighter.

"I'd say no, but you might keep yours longer than normal. Do your best to exercise, eat, and rest while your body deals with side effects of the chemo. On day fourteen, you'll have a bone marrow biopsy—a big day."

"That's coming up the end of the week isn't it?" Doug said.

"I think that's right. I'll check."

"If the doctors see the results they want, we'll be able to reschedule the transplant?" I sat on the bed next to Doug.

"That's the plan. Just keep doing what you're doing and cross your fingers." The nurse moved toward the door. "Let me know if either of you need anything."

My phone rang. I followed her out into the hallway to keep from disturbing Doug.

"Hi Mom. How's Doug doing?" It was Jill. "I checked on CaringBridge and it sounded like he'd finished chemo and tolerated it well."

"This is one time I don't mind repeating myself. Today looks like it'll be just like yesterday. He's got energy, is eating well and in good spirits."

"Oh, I'm so glad. We've been praying like crazy. You'd be surprised how many prayer warriors are on Doug's team."

"Thanks for spreading the word. Please pass on our gratitude." Tears welled in my eyes. "He's watching a golf tournament and squeezing on a grip-strengthening device."

"Sounds like the normal Papa."

"How are the kids? We really miss them. Please tell them thanks for the artwork they send."

"Kids are fine. They miss you too. Seems like someone is always coughing and sniffling, so we don't want to come visit."

"I wish you could come, but we need to be safe. It's so far with your busy schedule just to wave at him through the window of the door."

"Take care, Mom. Tell Papa we love him and miss him."

Stop! I Want to Get Off

The next morning, I blinked and blinked trying to wake up. Morning light filtered through the blinds. I checked my watch. How could it be 6 a.m.? I slept seven hours right through nurses coming in and out of the room, flipping on the lights to take vitals and draw blood. That must be a hospital record. I looked over at Doug who was scratching like crazy.

"What's up honey?"

"Boy, you slept like a rock. I'm fine, except for this horrible rash. It's everywhere. I can't stop digging at it. The nurse said she'd ask the doctor for something to relieve it."

On cue, the nurse brought him a pill. After a few minutes, Doug settled down. The rash remained and looked awful. I worked hard to keep myself from clawing at it for him.

"I'll be right back. I'm going to the restroom. Would you please ask the nurse for a cup of coffee with lots of cream if one stops by?"

When I got back, no sign of the nurse but food service had been there. I smelled bacon as I entered the room. Doug tackled breakfast with a good appetite. I folded my bedding and put it away.

"How are you doing?" A nurse breezed in. "Has the medicine helped?"

"The rash still looks terrible, but the itching stopped almost immediately." I spoke up for Doug since he had a mouthful of eggs.

"Great, so glad to hear that. The doctor was puzzled about the itching. Chemo often causes rashes, but typically, they don't itch. Doctor Aljitawi thinks you might be reacting to the platelets we gave you yesterday. From now on, we'll give you Benadryl if you need more platelets. I'll be back in a few minutes with the results of this morning's blood draw. Can I get you anything?"

"I'd love a cup of coffee, if you're not too busy."

"You like lots of cream, don't you?"

"Sure do. How nice you remembered." I smiled.

The nurse returned with coffee and the latest news. As expected, Doug's white count dropped in response to the chemo. His temperature and other vitals were normal. His oxygen level remained at 100%. Doug did not have many red blood cells, but the ones he had must be working hard.

"Oh Doug, I pray you continue to tolerate treatment this well. I saw the doctor in the hallway. He said you probably won't lose your hair until the third week. Just think, then you won't have to shave."

"Oh brother, aren't you're in a good mood? I'll be weirdly bald, and you see a silver lining."

Over the next few days, the rash continued, but it didn't bother him. His appetite was good. What a blessing to see him eating scrambled eggs, French toast, yogurt, and fruit cups. That afternoon we noticed a new rash around the dressing on his arm. I rang for the nurse.

"This is going to sting like the devil. I'm going to have to yank it off and clean the area."

"Just do it quickly." Doug closed his eyes.

I cringed and steeled myself against more torture for my poor husband. He didn't scream or grimace.

"Are you doing okay?" The nurse glanced at him as she began cleaning the area.

"That wasn't bad at all. It actually feels better now that you're cleaning it."

"That's great, but surprising." The nurse shook her head.

The area looked terrible. The nurse noted the allergy in his chart. She instructed us to remind anyone who changed his dressing he needed hypoallergenic bandages.

When the doctor made his rounds, Doug asked him if the rash would disappear. He assured us it would. The area effected by Doug's reaction to the dressing didn't bother him, but it was the reddest rash I had ever seen.

Since Doug was doing well, I left him to run some errands, work a little, and help Jean with deliveries for KC Quality Products. He seemed blue, but swore he was fine with me leaving. I probably projected my mood onto him.

€€€

The following day when I returned, Doug was tired and sleepy. No slacker, he managed to get four fifteen-minute walks around the hall anyway. I was constantly amazed at his tenacity. Just as Doug finished his walk, the doctor came in to examine him. Doug perked right up.

"You're our star patient, and I have some good news for you. Once the leukemia is in remission, you can go home for two weeks. During that time, you can eat anything and do whatever you want."

"What?" Doug and I said in unison.

"That's right. On Friday, we'll take another biopsy to find out if you're in remission. If you are, you'll recoup for a couple of weeks, possibly three here in the hospital. Then another bone marrow biopsy. If you're still in remission, you'll go home."

Doug and I looked at each other. Tears slid down my cheeks, and Doug's smile was the biggest I had seen in a long time. We shook the doctor's hand and thanked him profusely. What joy to see the doctor's grin after all the somber expressions we'd seen on his face.

€€€

Since I continued to caution everyone about how careful they needed to be about visiting, we remained isolated. One evening, I was shocked to look up and see my college roommate, Sherry, and her husband, Allan, walk through the door of Doug's room unannounced. I jumped up and threw my arms around Sherry. Doug enjoyed their visit although he stayed at the opposite side of the room.

We laughed, joked, and life felt normal. I hoped this would be the start of regular drop-ins. It felt like solitary confinement was over. That visit coupled, with the doctor's news that Doug could go home for two weeks, filled me with a hope I hadn't been able to find for a long time.

€€€

I had always loved roller coasters, but the one we rode now made a boring merry-go-round extremely appealing. I forgot the day's good news at 9 pm when I noticed Doug looked terrible. I thought he was exhausted from all his trips up and down the hall. He pushed himself beyond reason, eager to get to the two-week reprieve. He had been restless last night, but this was different.

Doug touched his neck gingerly and mentioned his throat was sore. I knew that wasn't good. I touched his forehead, and it felt warm. I panicked and hustled to get the nurse.

She came immediately and took his temperature. It was approaching the worry zone of 100.5 degrees.

"I'll be in frequently to monitor his temp."

In no time, it rose to 103 degrees. Doug shook the whole bed with his chills.

The nurse sprang into action. She reinserted IVY, drew blood for cultures, and administered new antibiotics, fluids, and Tylenol. Typically, the nurses were chatty, explained what they were doing, and answered questions. I always had questions. Now it was different. This nurse was quiet. I didn't say a word. Her need to concentrate on Doug was palpable.

She hurried toward the door. "I'm going to let the doctor on call know what's going on. I'll be right back." Minutes later, she rushed back in with ice packs. She turned down the room temperature and piled on the ice. His temperature was not going down. She brought in a cool blanket and placed it under him.

Doug didn't complain of the cold. He was too busy shivering. I stayed out of her way, and kept silent, not to distract her. But my brain exploded with questions. Horrified, all I could do was watch him shiver and moan as he tossed and turned. He opened his eyes, and I felt his misery.

He begged, "Evie, please pray for me. Please pray for me."

Nighttime makes things scarier, and all this went on in the semi-darkness of his room. My fear ramped up with every minute that passed. Each time the nurse took his temperature, we hoped it would be lower. Finally, it slowly receded.

Relief relaxed her expression, and her frantic pace slowed. "This has been frightening for both of you, but it's quite normal with chemo patients. The doctor ordered Ativan to help Doug sleep."

I did my best to believe her as I thought about asking for some Ativan of my own. I dozed a bit, but spent most of the night thanking God it was over. Doug had been in serious trouble. I don't care how normal these events are for chemo patients. He was blessed to have survived and I was full of gratitude the nurse was so conscientious and competent.

In the morning, his temperature was 101.3 degrees. Yesterday that would have been frightening. Today it sounded wonderful. He slept peacefully.

One of our favorite nurses came in with a worried look instead of her normal cheerful one. "I hear Doug had a rough night."

Doug managed to open his eyes. "It was horrible."

"Though last night was awful, it's quite common. It's not a question of will it happen, but when will it happen."

"We had visitors last night. I'll bet I caught it from them." Doug closed his eyes again.

I shook my head. "Honey, they couldn't cause you to get sick that fast."

The nurse assured Doug. "Your wife is right. It couldn't happen that fast. Actually, most infections come from the patient's skin."

"Maybe, but I don't want to risk that happening again. No more visitors."

I sank in my chair. His fear didn't make sense, but I would respect his wishes. I put the word out on CaringBridge. No more visitors.

Since Doug was exhausted and finally able to sleep, I left the room. I asked the nurse to call my cell when the doctors arrived for morning rounds.

I took the elevator down to the lovely little café in the Heart Center. They had a Starbucks, an unnecessary luxury, but I enjoyed a Tall Skinny Vanilla Latte every chance I got. Last night justified a Grande. I had nearly filled my punch card and would soon get a free drink.

Since I couldn't get to my toothpaste, hairbrush, or soap without disturbing Doug, I looked like a homeless person hanging out at the hospital among the morning crowd of dress-up clothes, perfect ponytails, and the bright eyes of those who had slept last night.

Fatigue spared me from feeling too embarrassed by my uncombed hair, baggy sweats and one bare foot in my tennis shoe. Somehow, I had lost the other sock. It seemed impossible to lose anything in that tiny space. I was sure it would turn up, but it was quite an annoyance and added to my disheveled look. My kingdom for a sock.

Spending time in the coffee shop revived me. When I left Doug's room, I managed to grab my computer. I finished a project for work and felt like part of the outside world again. The nurse called just as I snapped my computer closed. The doctors were nearing Doug's room.

I hustled upstairs in time to meet them at the door. Our conversation roused Doug. He blinked his eyes and lay there docile and weak. The doctor donned his stethoscope and listened to his heart.

Dr. Aljitawi finished his exam and looked at Doug. "I'm sorry to hear you had such a rough night. You have an infection, and we're working on its source. You still have a low-grade fever, and your wife told us you have no appetite."

"I have no energy, don't feel like eating, and I've got an awful headache."

"We can take care of that. I'll have the nurse give you something. You're doing well, even though you don't feel like it. We're pleased with your tolerance of treatment. Get some rest and try to eat something."

The nurse gave Doug some medicine for the headache. He immediately fell back to sleep for several hours. I read a book and wrote an entry on CaringBridge until he awoke.

"Hi. Sleepy head. Hope you feel better." I said with a cheerfulness I didn't feel.

"What time is it?" Doug opened his eyes and shifted his head on the pillow.

"It's nearly 5 o'clock."

"Seriously? I slept almost all day?"

"Why not, after the night you had? I'm sick to my stomach you had to go through that." My resolve to be upbeat oozed away. "They were worried, no matter what they say. I've never seen a nurse work so quickly and intensely. I hope that fever is over, and you can get your strength back. Are you hungry?"

"I think I can eat something."

"Great! How about a protein shake?"

"Yeah, vanilla."

I walked out to the nurses' station and ordered his shake. The nurse brought it right away. He drank the whole thing.

"I feel really grubby."

"I bet you do after that high fever. You tossed and turned enough to feel like you'd run a marathon."

"I feel strong enough to shower."

"I'll get some help in case you need it. Besides, someone has to disconnect IVY."

"Okay, but I don't need anyone standing around in the bathroom. I'm not helpless."

"I understand, but please call me if you feel too weak. I'll get someone to change your linens too."

After his shower, Doug fell into bed, and I covered him up. He looked clean and cozy.

"It looks like you're ready for another nap. I'm going home to shower, do laundry, mail, and other stuff. Since it's so late, I'll stay home and see you in the morning."

"Sure, don't rush back, I'm fine." He drifted off to sleep as I gathered my things.

€€€

When I walked into his room the next morning, Doug looked like his old self. The nurse told me he ate a good breakfast and took his fifteen-minute walk in the hall. He sat in the recliner reading.

Of course, I was thrilled to see him that way, but I suffered emotional whiplash from all the jerky ups and downs his treatment caused. I was ready for some steady improvement.

I gave him a big hug. "Has the doctor been in yet?"

"No, I'm glad you didn't miss him."

We heard a knock on the door. Doctor Aljitawi walked in grinning. "The lab has determined your PICC was the source of the infection. The IV team will remove it and insert a new one today. Also, I have some excellent news for you."

"We could use it." Doug sat up.

"Lie back. You need to take it easy," The doctor said.

"Back to the good news. What is it?" I stared at him.

"Now, I caution you, these are only preliminary findings, but I called the pathologist to see if he had the results of your latest bone marrow biopsy.

"And?" I put both hands over my mouth.

"He said there was nothing—no cancer. We have to wait until Monday for the results to be final."

"Oh my gosh! Does this mean in two weeks, Doug can go home?" I asked.

"Probably, but don't hold me to two weeks exactly. Depends how quickly Doug can coax his bone marrow to produce good cells. Could take longer." He pointed his finger at us. "He'll need another bone marrow biopsy to confirm he's clean—no cancer cells. That would mean he's in remission. Then he can go home. The clinic will keep close tabs on him. Congratulations!"

"Thank you, Doc, and thank you, God." Doug's eyes teared up, and he shook his head. "I can't believe it. I could be going home in a few weeks."

"I need to warn you that most likely you'll be plagued by fevers off and on for the next ten days or so while your bone marrow gets its act together."

"I can handle that as long as it's not as bad as it was two nights ago." Doug's face drooped.

"It won't be. We're going to get this infection under control right away. Then we can watch for your blood values to rise. Once they start going up, it could progress rapidly, so don't get discouraged."

ƐƐƐ

Doug slept well that night, no doubt dreaming of going home. In the morning, he walked the hall for fifteen minutes and took a shower. After he exercised a little more in his room, he ate a small breakfast. Notable feats for one who had been so fatigued. He drifted off for a nap.

I left the room to walk the halls and get some breakfast. I made some phone calls and browsed at the gift shop. Time slipped away. When I checked my watch, I had been gone over two hours. I hurried upstairs to check on Doug. He was still asleep.

For the first time since I had known Doug, I wondered if I might have to force him to exercise. He needed to walk and eat. I hoped he'd get his energy back soon. It's not my nature to crack the whip. I wanted to let Doug sleep. I walked into the hall and stopped one of the nurses. "What's the minimum amount of walking Doug needs to do daily? He's so tired."

"It's fine for him to rest for a couple of days. This part of treatment is difficult. He needs to try to eat though. Even if it's just the protein shakes. He'll feel better soon, maybe even tomorrow."

"I hope so. Thanks."

Hope on the Horizon

The next morning, we learned one of Doug's meds made him extra tired, achy and cranky. He didn't have to take it anymore. Yay!

The doctor and his team came by while Doug ate biscuits and gravy with gusto.

"Keep eating, don't let us interrupt. That's important. I'm happy to tell you your WBC is up to .5 and we were able to count 10 neutrophils. Would you like to name them?"

"Sure," Doug said. "We have ten grandkids. Let's go with that."

Doctor Aljitawi laughed. "Perfect. You have to build those ten into close to five hundred and then you can go home."

I groaned. "Five hundred. That's a long way from ten."

"It sounds like it, but once they start, they really take off. This is excellent news. You're headed in the right direction." He patted Doug's shoulder. "Your body is on its way. The days will steadily get better. But…"

I interrupted "There will be ups and downs."

He frowned at me. "Yes, there will. That's the nature of this complicated cure."

Just after the good-news doctor left, a nurse came in with a bunch of mail. Balloons from Doug's cousins, cards from his niece and nephew. Best of all, several art pieces from the grandkids.

€€€

As he gradually regained his strength, Doug used part of his energy to be irritable and grumpy. The nurses understood and were accommodating. He remained stiff and slow over the next few days, but I saw hints of him being more himself. His appetite improved. He was more gracious when he made his wishes known, and directed the nurses and aides to do things his way. "Please put my arm in a plastic bag. Don't wrap it with Saran Wrap. Get some plastic bags and rubber bands. I don't want to shower today."

I saw a few eye rolls, but the whole staff was remarkably tolerant. It takes a thick skin to care for cancer patients who feel awful much of the time.

Each day we waited for the results of his blood draw, holding our breaths as the nurse walked in with the report. His white count crept up slightly to .6. We reminded each other what the doctor said. "We're headed in the right direction."

"Jamie's coming to town for a visit. She found cheap plane tickets for the girls and herself. I told her the girls could make funny faces at you through the windows in the doors at the end of the hall, but they can't come in."

"We need to make sure Jamie isn't sick. Now that I'm so close, I couldn't handle a setback that kept me from going home."

"I understand, and I'll be very clear with her. She really wants to see you. It's been hard on her being so far away. I'm over the moon at the idea of seeing them."

The next day, Jamie called me. "We're in the lobby. Can you come get us?"

I made it in record time. I swept our granddaughters, six-year-old Penelope and four-year-old Amelia into my arms and drank in their hugs and giggles. Jamie held me tight for a long moment.

"Oh, I'm so glad to see you. Is everyone healthy?"

"Yep."

We went to a couch where we could snuggle. "Papa has to be very careful of germs. He can't see you girls because of the hospital rules. You have to be twelve to get in, so only Josh is old enough."

Penelope, our serious one, looked a bit worried and confused.

Amelia looked around the lobby and spied the cafe. "Can we have hot chocolate?"

"You bet! As soon as we take Mom up to see Papa. He'll come to the window, so you can say hi."

"Let's go see Papa." Amelia said and jumped up.

Penelope stood and held my hand. "Papa is okay honey. He just needs to be safe from germs. Don't worry."

We took the elevator to the fourth floor. I called Doug to meet us at the door. He was there when we arrived. Both the girls tentatively walked close to the door. They didn't lose their serious looks until Papa smiled and waved. They returned smiles and waves, but stepped back quickly when Jamie opened the door to enter.

I took them for a walk around the hospital while Jamie had some time with Doug. We stopped at the coffee shop and indulged in not only a hot chocolate, but a pastry as well. Amelia was in heaven. Being with them renewed my soul and reminded me of the good stuff in the outside world. I was anxious for Doug to participate in that part of life, even for two weeks. It made such a difference to escape the small realm of the hospital.

Jamie met us in the lobby. "Doug seems frail and tired, but he has a great attitude. I'm happy to see that. We had a good visit. I didn't know what to expect. I'm glad I came."

"I am too. I know it was good for him. The girls and I had a great time." I teared up.

Jamie hugged me tightly. "Mom, I can't imagine how hard this has been for you. I wish I lived closer."

"Me too."

"I need to get the girls settled. It's been a long day. I'll see you tomorrow."

€€€

A week later, I came down with a virus. The doctor banned me from seeing Doug. For the time being, I picked up his dirty clothes and brought clean ones. An aide met me at the fourth floor elevator for the exchange. I couldn't even wave at Doug through the unit door. To make matters worse, he had fevers again. He felt so lousy, some days he didn't even want to talk to me on the phone.

On those days, I called the unit and talked to the nurse. "Doug is having a bit of a rough time again. He's had to have extra antibiotics and transfusions to keep up his platelets and HGB. Don't worry, this is common."

"It's so discouraging. Both of us expected more improvement by now. These fevers really take him down. I'm feeling better. I hope I can come see him soon."

"I'm sure that would help you both. Take care of yourself. He's doing fine."

"It's hard to believe he's still on track to come home soon." I shook my head.

"Don't worry, he is."

With his constantly-changing condition, it was difficult to imagine he was doing fine. Homecoming seemed forever away. He spiked fever after fever.

When I called him after three days of not seeing him, I could barely hear him as he whispered. "These fevers are horrible. I don't feel like doing anything. I can't read the books Gin and Kay sent or even check emails."

"These fevers have to be over soon." It was hard to be a cheerleader when I couldn't believe my own slogans. "At least the Red Wings are doing their part. They're headed to the playoffs. Those games give you a lot to look forward to."

"I guess. Are you getting better? When do you think you can come and see me?"

"I'm feeling much better, and I'm going to check in with the doctor. I'll let you know as soon as I find out."

"I miss you."

"Miss you too."

I hung up and called the nurses' station. "What's going on with Doug? He sounds really down."

"He is. On top of not feeling good because of the fevers, his temperature appears to be burning up his platelets. He ran 100 degrees, not a big deal. But his platelets are low, and he's going to have more again today. The doctor has ordered cross matching in case Doug has developed antibodies and that's what's destroying them. Obviously, something's going on."

"I don't understand what all this means. It doesn't sound like he's getting better."

"It's frustrating but trust the doctors. They aren't worried. I'll give you the numbers, but that may cause even more confusion. His WBC is up to .7. That's the highest it's been."

"Oh good, but that's moving up at a snail's pace. What about his neutrophils? That seems like the number that matters most."

"We don't have that yet."

I slumped and sighed. "Okay thanks. I'll call Doug later. Maybe by then you'll have it."

When I talked to Doug later, he was angry. "What's the deal? Every time they weigh me, it's different. One time I'm 163 pounds and then next I'm 186. I've never weighed 186 pounds in my life."

"Honey, it doesn't really matter does it?"

"Of course it does! My medication dosages depend on it."

"Good point. I'll talk to the nurse about it."

"I already did. If they can't get it right, you're gonna have to bring a scale, for Pete's sake."

It was good to hear a strong voice from him even if he was upset. He had been so tired and weak lately.

"I have to go. My breakfast is here." He hung up.

On Wednesday, I was able to talk to the nurse practitioner. "How's Doug doing?"

"Unbelievably well. He sailed through this process. If he continues to do this well, he'll probably do the same with the transplant."

Really? He sailed through? She must be thinking of the wrong patient. With all the miserable problems he had, I'd hate to see what not sailing through looked like. I'm going with her positive attitude. Why not? "I'm glad to hear that." I didn't have the energy to question her.

"The doctor is pleased that his platelets held steady after a night of no fever. He's not developing antibodies against them."

"I assume that's good, though I don't completely understand."

"Yes, that's good. It means his fevers were burning them up, and it could also mean that his bone marrow is making some of his own platelets."

"Now those are words I understand. That's part of what we've been waiting for. Right?"

"Right. Yesterday his neutrophils were 60, and we expect good results again today. Doctor Ganguly said by Friday, the team would have a good idea of his progress and probably be able to give him a tentative date for going home. Remember, that's a tentative date."

"I'll take that. I guess he has to have another bone marrow biopsy too."

"That shouldn't be a problem."

Back Together

Finally, on Friday, the doctor cleared me. I couldn't wait to call Doug. "Hey guess what? Ganguly told me it's safe for me to visit again."

"That's great. Can't wait to see you. Gotta go. My eggs are getting cold." Click.

He sounded like himself, as if I were talking to him at the office. Apparently, he had his appetite back. I hurried to get ready and left for the hospital. The nurses had warned me he would be swollen and discolored. I was prepared for a purple balloon boy and Doug did not disappoint. I didn't care what he looked like. I just wanted to be with him. Though it was only a few days, it felt like a month.

€€€

Each morning, we waited for the results of Doug's blood test. We jumped up when we saw the nurse come in with the report.

"How are they today?" Doug raised his eyebrows.

"They're going in the right direction. The doctors are pleased."

We wilted back into our chairs. Good news certainly, but we longed for something concrete.

"Why is this going so slow? I don't understand. The docs act all excited, but I want that next bone marrow biopsy now. I want it to be clean. I want to go home!" Doug said.

"Just think—when it happens you can eat anything you want, go anywhere you want, and see the kids." I moved over to sit on the side of his bed.

"Just think? Are you kidding? It's all I can think about. I dream about it day and night. I can't wait to see the kids. I hope they're healthy, or I'll be nervous after all this caution. I want McDonald's French fries. I want to sit in my recliner, sleep in my bed. It's impossible to say everything going home means to me." He flopped back on his pillow. I thought he was going to cry.

That wasn't the only unknown driving us crazy. They told us the rescheduled transplant would take place sometime in May. But when?

Doctor Aljitawi surprised us when he poked his head in the door since he had already been in earlier during rounds. "Are you awake?"

"Sure, what's up?" Doug said.

The doctor settled on the chair next to Doug's bed. Obviously, he had something out of the ordinary to say, but I couldn't read his face. Was it good or bad?

"All the uncertainty and waiting must be very difficult for you. It's also challenging the donor to be on call for such an unpredictable timetable. More importantly, you need the transplant when you're ready before the blasts start production again. We have a very small window." He put his elbows on his knees and clasped his hands as he leaned forward.

I gasped. "Small window? What are you telling us?"

"After you come back to the hospital in a couple of weeks, you'll start the pre-transplant chemo. We have to do the transplant within two days of the last dose of chemo. We have no time for donor glitches."

"Oh no! What does that mean?" I turned to Doug.

"Evie, settle down so we can hear what the doctor has to say."

The doctor smiled. "You're okay. Don't worry. We've asked the donor to schedule his part of the process. The extracted cells will be sent to KU to be frozen until Doug needs them."

I looked to the heavens, "Oh thank God there's a way to fix it. I don't think I could take one more thing to worry about."

Doug sighed. "No kidding. It feels so good to know the cells will be here. I don't need any more scheduling disasters."

€€€

Doug's blood levels improved. Finally, it was time for the bone marrow biopsy that could send him home.

Thursday, the team came in for rounds. "Doug you're doing very well." Doctor Aljitawi said. "In fact, unless something comes up, you can go home next Monday. The biopsy results should be in by then."

Late Friday evening, Doctor Aljitawi stuck his head in the door. "I know you're anxiously waiting to hear, and I just got an unofficial result." He grinned as he walked in the door. "You're going home next week."

I burst into tears, grabbed Doug and held him close. "Thank you, oh thank you."

My husband freed himself from my hug and stepped forward. He shook Doctor Aljitawi's hand. Doug's Adam's apple bobbed as he tried to swallow his emotions. "Thanks for letting me know. Monday felt like forever away."

"That's his birthday," I choked out.

"Really? Great timing. Congratulations."

"Thanks Doc. I've never had a better birthday gift. I can't imagine ever coming close."

He examined Doug, then headed for the door. "I'll see you tomorrow. Enjoy your afternoon."

"You'll have a birthday cake this year after all," I said. "I'll get you anything you want."

"I'll take an ice cream cake from Dairy Queen," he said licking his lips.

I hid my doubts from Doug. Despite Doctor Aljitawi's good news, it was difficult to imagine he would be eating birthday cake at home on his 63rd birthday. His skin looked purple and itchy and he had swelling in his hands, legs, ankles, and feet.

Happy Birthday Doug

No more glitches. Doug was set free on his birthday, May 6th. The prospect of two whole weeks of being normal again filled us with joy and optimism.

A nurse came in to give us our discharge instructions. "It's a perfect spring day out there— a great day to be going home."

"That's cool," Doug said. "But any day would be a great day to go home."

A tear slipped from my eye as I continued to pack our things.

The nurse handed Doug some papers to sign. "I've called transportation, and they should be here any minute. Then as soon as we go over the papers, you can leave. You'll be following up with the clinic tomorrow. They'll keep a close eye on you."

"Go get the van." Doug ordered. "I didn't mean to be so brusque, but it'll take you awhile. I can't wait to get out of here. Take what you can manage. I'll hold the rest in my lap. Even though I can walk just fine, I guess I'm stuck riding in a wheelchair."

"See you soon." I rushed out of the room. I hurried across the street and up the elevator to the top deck of the parking garage. The antiseptic smell of hand cleaner and alcohol wipes disappeared from my nostrils, forced away by the sweet fragrance of all the spring blossoms mixed together. Since my countless trips back and forth to the hospital blended, I always parked in the same area. It was especially important today. No time to wander around trying to remember where the van was. Doug would be waiting anxiously at the main entrance.

In a few moments, Doug would be rid of the hospital sights, sounds, smells, and routine with all its poking and prodding. I circled down the parking garage ramps and drummed my fingers on the steering wheel as I waited in line to pay. I pulled up in front of the main entrance.

Doug saw me, sprang from the wheelchair, and dove into the passenger seat. The nurse smiled and helped me load the rest of our possessions.

"I can't believe I'm sitting in my van. I wish I could drive."

"I wish you could too. I can't wait for you to see the tulips blooming everywhere in the Plaza."

I drove toward The Country Club Plaza, an outdoor shopping area just a few minutes from the hospital. The Plaza touted upscale stores, hotels, offices, and restaurants. Its architecture modeled a Seville, Spain theme. Fountains and artistic tile work made it a great place to stroll, whether shopping or sightseeing. It covered about fifty-five acres from forty-fifth to fifty-first between Broadway and Madison. The landscaping was gorgeous, a beautiful place to visit any time of year.

Christmastime Plaza lights are famous, a part of Kansas City tradition since 1930. The Christmas season officially begins on Thanksgiving night when 80 miles of lights with 280,000 multi-colored bulbs catapult the Plaza into a magical place. Thousands of people crowd the area to begin their holiday season. The lights remain until the middle of January. Though I love the Plaza lights, its spring blooms are my favorite.

I don't know if tulips have a fragrance, but the sheer volume of them packed onto every median tricked my senses into believing they did. I had seen them many times as I ferried back and forth to the hospital. But to share it with my husband was a completely different experience.

I could barely keep my eyes on the road as I glanced at Doug. His face was full of wonder like a man whose sight had been restored. I blinked my eyes to push away tears, but this time their source was joy.

Doug opened his window. "Listen to the birds. Look at that sunshine and all those blossoms. The colors and smells.... I didn't know if I'd be a part of the world outside my hospital room ever again." His voice caught.

I couldn't imagine a better route home after a month-long view of black rooftops. "Do you want to stop and get something to eat or walk around a little?"

"No, I just want to get home. Any kind of food that doesn't come from the hospital sounds great, but I'm actually craving McDonald's French Fries. I can smell them already. Let's pick some up and get home."

He walked through our front door like a soldier returning from war. He dropped his bags and glanced around. "I can't believe I'm here. I'll be sleeping in my own bed with nobody waking me to take blood. Showering in my own bathroom. No nurse just outside the door asking me if everything is okay. I can't wait to sit in my recliner and read."

I couldn't contain my tears and let them run down my cheeks. We hugged and thanked God, but only briefly. The smell of McDonald's Fries called to him. He sat at the kitchen table, savored them, and looked out into the backyard, smiling at the pesky squirrels digging up the lawn.

"What are you thinking?"

"I'm imagining the day I can take over the yardwork."

Our neighbor had been mowing for us and refused to let us pay him.

"Did you get some gift cards for Ted? We can't let him do all that work indefinitely."

"I forced him to take some restaurant gift cards, but I'll find a more permanent solution. It may be a while until you can do all you used to do."

His smile faded. "You're right."

After he stuffed himself with fries, Doug went to the bedroom to unpack. He opened the drawers in his dresser. "I can't tell you how good it is to put these clothes away, to be here with all my stuff. I'm going to organize my books and other things. Then I'll make a list of all the things I want to eat and do in the next two weeks."

"I'm going to get your birthday cake. Still want Dairy Queen?"

"I do, but I'm tired. As much as I want to see family, let's keep it to just you and me."

"This has been a big day. I think that's a smart decision."

€€€

Though we continued to be cautious of anyone with signs of illness, we went to family gatherings and hit the restaurant circuit hard. The grandkids were beyond happy to see Papa. They were afraid to hug him or get too close. I coaxed the little ones to hug his leg.

Doug and I frequented the clinic for checkups. Each time, they confirmed he was doing great. We called those visits our doctor dates and always stopped for breakfast or lunch. Doug was his old self.

Other than a few inconveniences, life at home was wonderful. The three color-coded lumens for his PICC required daily flushing. My independent husband liked to do everything himself, but this was not a one-handed job. I added it to my—I never thought I could do this—list. We did it together, and Doug watched me closely. I don't think he trusted me. It was hard to keep track of which one to do next even though they were different colors. As I completed the red one, he would hold the white one out for me. We both announced the color aloud as we finished it.

When he showered, we had to wrap his arm in a plastic bag we'd cut open at the bottom and secure it with rubber bands to keep it completely dry. The PICC was a daily reminder of what was to come.

Those two weeks flew by faster than any other fourteen days in our lives. Doug felt wonderful and life was normal. Why couldn't it end here? Why couldn't those nasty cancer blasts stop multiplying, and leave him alone?

Fantasizing didn't alter reality. The doctors assured us, the cells would be back. And without the transplant, those cells would kill him.

€€€

After about ten days at home, Doug wanted to write his own entry on CaringBridge:

"Hi Everyone! Doug here. It's Wednesday, May 15th, 6:30 pm in Independence, MO. Evie and I just finished a great home-cooked meal. We ate off real plates, at a real kitchen table, with real tableware, while looking out at real trees and real grass. It's amazing what you appreciate after spending four weeks in a small hospital room. Hospital rooms, beds, food, and nurses are tolerable for a week. After that, it becomes a real test. Prison life easily comes to mind. I can't tell you how good it feels to be back in the real world.

"Sometime next week I'll go back to the hospital for the main event: chemo and the bone marrow transplant. I'm nervous of course, but I'm truly grateful modern medicine has progressed to the point where there is hope for people in my predicament. Speaking of gratitude, Evie and I recognize how hugely blessed we've been by all of you. Both of us are humbled by the support that has come our way. Everyone who has sent well wishes, cards, gifts, and thoughts feels like part of the team that is helping me through this challenge. I feel for anyone who has to go through anything like this alone.

"I don't believe I can ever thank you for all you've done for us. We are truly grateful. I haven't forgotten the donor. Somewhere, a twenty-six-year old man has made a decision to donate his life-giving cells so I can have, God willing, the chance to extend my life. I'd love to play hockey til I'm 85.

"This next stay in the hospital will be a challenge. I'm going to give it everything I've got. I hope my efforts are worthy of all the love, concern and support that you, my teammates, have sent my way. Thank you so much."

Room 4109

It was time to return to the 4th Floor at KU. Doug packed up, determined to fight for his life with whatever it took. He brought clothes, because he still refused to wear a hospital gown except at the nurses' insistence for a particular procedure. He also carried a boom box, lots of reading material, snacks and a great attitude.

This time I'd be in the right place when I entered Unit 41 through the airlock door. The unit had only twelve rooms. The purpose of the airlock system and careful scrutiny before visitors could enter was to protect against germs. All the patients in various stages of pre and post transplant were highly susceptible to infections of all kinds.

Doug's new home for the next thirty days was straight down the hall in Room 4109. We walked in and dropped our baggage.

"Oh my gosh!" Doug turned to me with wide eyes.

"Look at this. I can't believe it. It's like a resort hotel room." He spun around in disbelief. "This room is more than twice as big as my prison cell. Look at that huge window. I see blue skies, trees, cars, and people. A pigeon just landed on the outside ledge."

We both pumped our fists and cheered.

"Looks like you have plenty of space for nervous pacing." I joined him at the window. "The outside hall is T-shaped, but big enough for your daily walk."

We settled in to begin the countdown to the transplant. The next morning, day minus six, chemo started. Doug was on a regular diet until day minus two, so he skipped the hospital breakfast. He wanted a blueberry muffin from Starbucks. I felt as if I was smuggling in contraband. I quickly closed the door in deference to the patients who were on a neutropenic diet.

After two days of chemo, Doug was feeling fine. When the team came in for morning rounds, Doug greeted them. "Hey Doc, can I get a stationary bike for my room?"

"That would be great. We used to have one, but no one ever used it. I don't know what happened to it. Exercise is extremely important." Doctor Aljitawi turned to the other team members and smiled. "Most of the time we have to persuade patients to get up and walk the hall. In Doug's case, we have to caution him not to overdo."

I saw Doug's wheels start to turn. He was all over the internet researching the best tool for the job. He found exactly what he wanted, called the bike shop, and bought it with his credit card.

"When can you pick it up for me? I really need to get my hands on it and start exercising."

"Let me check with the kids so I can get some help."

€€€

The next day I went to lunch with my college roommate, Jeanne. I explained to her how obsessed Doug was about getting the bike. "I'm a little afraid he'll make a break for it and head to the bike shop."

She grinned. "Let's go get it, and take it to him."

"Really? I'd love that. Do you think we can manage it by ourselves? I was going to ask Matt or Joel, but they're always so busy. I don't know when they'd get around to it."

"Let's do it right now. I've been looking for a way to help you and Doug."

We picked up the 100-pound high tech beauty at the bike shop. The owner helped us load it into the van. It looked like the two of us could manage it easily.

We parked directly in front of the hospital, in the area for unloading and loading of patients. I surprised myself with how persistent and persuasive I could be.

"You can't park here. What are you doing?" one of the attendants said.

I explained the situation. "Please let us park here just for a few moments to get the bike out and into the lobby."

He didn't budge. Another attendant walked over, and I pled my case. Finally, they agreed and even helped us get it out of the van.

"Make it quick. You need to get that vehicle out of here ASAP."

We wrestled our surprise through the hospital lobby, narrowly missing people as we struggled to travel a straight line with its stubborn wheels. It was like operating a heavy-duty power scrubber. Once you know how to work with it, it's a snap but when you fight it, it fights back.

People in the lobby gawked at us. It would have made a great World's Funniest Videos episode. We barged into the elevator. Passengers stared and stayed out of our way. Up to the fourth floor, down the hall and into the airlock room. We wiped it down with antiseptic wipes and battled our way into Room 4109.

Doug jumped out of the recliner. "What? How did you manage to get the bike here? I can't believe you did that. Jeanne, I can't thank you enough for helping Evie with this."

Jeanne grinned. "My pleasure. I'm happy to do whatever I can to help you through this. I hope you know that."

"I'll tell you one thing," I said, "If I'm responsible for getting this monster home, I'm donating it to the hospital. I need to run down and move the van. I'm parked illegally. Be right back."

"What do you mean? This bike is easy to move. What's the problem?" Doug flipped it over and rolled it easily with one hand guiding it.

Jeanne buckled over laughing.

I walked to the door. "If I ever get back to that bike shop, I'll give that owner a piece of my mind.

€€€

When Doug agreed to the clinical trial, he was randomly chosen to receive reduced chemo. The BMT team expected Doug to handle it well. He didn't disappoint. So far no nausea, vomiting, or other problems. He hadn't lost his hair as expected during his prior chemo treatment, but they assured us he would eventually lose his hair. It would likely grow back, maybe a different color or curly.

It was day minus three. "What would you like me to get you for your last meal?"

"Ugh, that's right. Tomorrow starts a month of hospital and packaged food. I'll have a Five Guys Burger, French fries and a vanilla shake."

I obliged happily, pleased he had a good appetite, in spite of feeling a bit tired. His mood was good. I thanked God every day for his attitude.

His doctors praised him for riding his bike and thanked him for providing inspiration for the other patients. When I stepped out into the hall to use the phone or walk, other BMT candidates asked me how Doug was doing.

It was time for his blood counts to drop, but they remained high. It drove me crazy to pray for his counts to go down. Three weeks ago my fervent prayers begged for his counts to go up.

I caught a doctor in the hallway. "I'm worried his counts won't drop low enough. Will that delay the transplant?"

"That's not a problem. Some of the longer living cells take a while to die, but they've been attacked by the chemo. Even after the chemo is out of Doug's body, they're marked for a slow death. They'll eventually die off."

During morning rounds the next day, Doug's good-natured woman doctor came to check on him. "You really are one of us. You've been a topic of discussion among the doctors. We were beginning to think you weren't human. Your blood count is finally dropping."

The next day, it was dark and quiet in Doug's room—a stark contrast from the usual bright lights and whir of the spinning bike wheel. Day minus two and no more Five Guys. Doug was on meds that made him sleepy. He wasn't interested in the hospital menu or much else except resting.

I reminded myself, we had to expect the complicated miracle of a bone marrow transplant would have some glitches. I went home from the hospital to do laundry, pay bills and sort mail that had piled up. The hospital was always farthest away when Doug called with bad news.

"The drug, Tacrolimus, the one to keep me from rejecting the donor cells, is giving me terrible hives. They gave me Benadryl and stopped the med. They tried again, and I got hives again. They tried a different drug and the hives were worse."

"I'll be there as soon as I can." I prayed there was another med he could tolerate and that they'd find it soon.

The doctors came in a minute after I arrived in Doug's room. "In fifteen years, no one has reacted like this to Tacrolimus. We'll try you on the oral version. Maybe you're allergic to something in the IV solution. You must take an anti-rejection drug for months after transplant. We have to find something."

Doug swallowed the Tacrolimus pill. As we waited to see his reaction, a cookie bouquet arrived from two of the Locker Room Angels. By the time he had unwrapped the gift, the critical twenty minutes had passed with no reaction.

Bingo! The oral med was okay. Praise God! It was crunch time. The transplant could not be delayed. Chemo had finished yesterday. It was necessary for the anti-rejection drug to be in Doug's system for twenty-four hours before he received the cells.

We were on schedule for the next day. Room 4109's door sported a decorated poster: "Happy Cell Day—May 29th."

The Main Event

"Today's the day, honey." I sighed and sat on Doug's bed. "I still don't know what to expect. I'll be so glad when it's over."

"It seems like I've waited forever for this, but I'm really nervous." Doug took a big breath.

There was a knock on the door. A nurse we'd never seen before entered with her hands full of giant syringes. They were bigger than cake decorating tubes. I heard Crocodile Dundee in the background. "Now *that's* a syringe."

"Hi, Douglas. I'm going to be giving you your cells. You've been pre-medicated with several medicines to help with side effects, but you may still experience dizziness, a warm sensation, and a bad taste. I brought you some mints because that bad taste is a very common complaint. Any questions?"

We shook our heads.

The nurse slowly pushed four syringes of life-saving cells into Doug's PICC line. He was dizzy, felt hot, and sucked on the mints for the bad taste. All minor things, which lasted only a short time. The main event was over quickly.

"Good luck. Be sure and let a nurse know if you experience any side effects or have questions," the nurse said and left the room.

"That was pretty anticlimactic." Doug opened another mint and popped it into his mouth. "I did feel weird, but at least there was no pain."

"It was totally underwhelming, but I'm so grateful. No more worries about something going wrong before you could get the cells. I feel like the day Beth's email said they had found your donor."

"Don't get too excited. It's only the beginning. We have a long road ahead of us."

"For sure, but it feels like we've started down the path to recovery instead of endlessly preparing for the journey." I grabbed my purse and stood. "I'm going to get a snack. I hate to leave you. I feel bad every time I leave the unit, knowing you can't."

"Quit that. Go! I'm happy you're not trapped like me. What's the point of us both being prisoners?"

"Do you want anything?"

"I'll take some candy."

I returned to Doug's room with lifesavers. "Yuck, does that smell bother you?"

"What smell?"

"I guess you're used to it. It smells like bad creamed corn. Glad it doesn't bother you. It makes me nauseous. I've crossed creamed corn off my food list permanently."

Doug screwed up his face and gave me a dirty look.

"Nothing personal and don't worry, I'll get used to it. I'm sure it won't last long."

Later, I found out frozen donor cells are known to smell like creamed corn due to the protective solution used when they are frozen.

€€€

During the next few days, the doctors and nurses reminded us of the precautions we would need to take at home. The chemo before the transplant destroyed Doug's immune system. That gave the donor's blood marrow cells the best chance to establish a new, healthy, cancer-free immune system. It was imperative that we protect his newborn immune system until it was well established.

I tried to talk to Doug about how careful we would need to be at home. He didn't appear to pay much attention to me. I couldn't blame him. It was daunting. Following the month in the hospital, if all went well, Doug would enter the infamous 100 days of extreme care. He would have to avoid pollen, dust, mold, and other contaminants.

I reminded him he could do only clean jobs like unloading the dishwasher, as opposed to dirty jobs like loading the dishwasher. I had my job cut out for me. I was destined to assume the position of Super Nag. The first few weeks at home would have loads of rules and medications. I was a wreck, worrying about keeping it all straight.

Doctor Abhyankar called the handful of meds Doug swallowed in the morning his pill breakfast. It would help prevent infections, rejection, and other side effects. I don't know how he choked it all down.

Though he didn't have to heal a painful wound from surgery, Doug faced many dangers: possible damage to his organs from the strong chemo, infections, and Graft versus Host Disease (GVHD). Any one of these could be serious or fatal. Regular side effects of chemo included hair loss, nausea and vomiting, mouth sores, and skin rash. Any one or all of them could show up at any time.

GVHD is an autoimmune disease. Directly after a transplant, acute GVHD is a positive side effect. It signifies that the donor cells are destroying any remaining cancer cells. Chronic GVHD is another story, which can cause a host of problems.

Bone marrow biopsies administered periodically would confirm engraftment, the process of donor cells taking over and creating Doug's new healthy immune system.

One day after lunch with Jeanne, I stopped to visit with the nurses. They had some good news. I hit the antibacterial gel machine, cleaned my hands in a hurry and rushed into Doug's room.

"I just found out that the days in the hospital after transplant count toward your 100 days."

"That's great!"

"Next time I go home, I'll bring the paper chains the kids made. You can start the countdown to normal again."

"I can't wait to get home, even though I won't be out of the woods until the magic 100 day mark. Surely I can gradually get back to my life."

"Just remember, we have to abide by the precautions"

"I'm sure you have them memorized."

"They seem to have more importance to me than to you. No casserole ministry...."

"What in the world does that mean?"

"Nobody can bring food over for us. Our church friends were organizing an effort to provide meals. What a bummer! We can't eat out, visitors are still limited, and your only outings will be to the clinic."

"Don't forget, I can't do dirty jobs." He mocked me.

"I don't care if you think that's overkill. I don't want you taking out the garbage, wiping up the kitchen floor, loading the dishwasher or cleaning the bathroom. I'd love the help but it's not worth taking the chance."

"Don't worry about it. I'm fine."

Those words made me crazy. They meant he wasn't going to stick to unloading the dishwasher or folding laundry. He was going to do whatever he wanted. "By the way, that 100 day goal isn't magic. The doctors will be keeping a close watch on you for at least six months."

"Don't remind me how long this will be. Right now 100 days is my focus."

"Don't forget, this won't be a picnic for me either. I have to cook everything. I was looking forward to help with meals."

"Honey, I know this is tough on you too. I appreciate all you've done, and all you'll still have to do. I just want to be my old self and do what I used to do."

"I didn't mean to make you feel bad. I can always make frozen food. I appreciate your willingness to eat simple meals. We'll get through this together."

My rah-rah comment didn't ring true in my mind, but I hoped I'd hidden that from Doug. I dreaded more isolation. Visitors would still have to be carefully screened and limited. He couldn't go to stores, restaurants, church, or any other public places. Because I couldn't leave him alone, the same rules applied to me. At home, there wouldn't be nurses and doctors. It would be even lonelier.

Preparations for Homecoming

Doug paced in his room. "I'm so antsy to know when I can go home."

"At least the 100 day clock has started ticking."

"Yeah that's good, but I wanna get out of here. I think Doctor Aljitawi said the quickest anyone left the hospital after transplant was twelve days. I'd sure like to break the record."

"I wouldn't be surprised if you did, but it's only been two days. Just in case, I better get busy. So much to do to get the house ready for your homecoming."

"Thanks for your concern, but don't work too hard."

I left the hospital with Doug doing well despite a little fatigue and nausea.

After driving home in a daze, I opened the front door and felt overwhelmed by all I needed to do. Somehow, I had to make this space a haven against pollen, dust, mold, and other contaminants. Luckily, we didn't have any pets or I would have had to find them foster homes.

I started a load of laundry and plopped down on the couch to make a list, but decided to do just a few things that night. I'd wait until morning to develop the masterplan. I banished plants to rooms Doug would inhabit least. I removed them from his bedroom and away from the couch in the family room. That was all I could manage. I took a bath and went to bed.

The next morning, dumbfounded with the responsibility of keeping Doug safe, I called out the troops. For months, family and friends offered help. It was time to tap the reservoir of those kind and caring folks.

I noticed I had a bit of a cough and worried I had a cold starting. It would be a good day to stay home and get stuff done. With help from my granddaughters, Emily and Chelsea, I removed the area rug from the family room. The hardwood floors would be easy to keep clean. We hauled it to the basement and unrolled it in a small sitting area.

"Wow Nonna!" (my grandma name) "That looks great down here," Emily said.

"It sure does. I think this should be its permanent home. I'll get a new one for the family room when Papa is better."

Back upstairs, I gave the girls a break while I dusted the floors, vacuumed the couches and Lazy Boy. Then together we scrubbed them down with antiseptic wipes. We removed most of the dust catchers and relegated the coffee table to the extra bedroom. Doug would have plenty of room for his stationary bike, the new focal point of our family room. That was enough for one day. The girls and I went out to eat, and I took them home.

It was late. I called Doug. "Honey, I'm going to stay home again tonight. How are you?"

"Good idea. I feel fine and you need the rest. Enjoy sleeping in your own bed. Soon I'll be able to do that."

"Have a good night. I don't know what time I'll be back to the hospital. Call me if you need anything."

"Okay. Good night."

Doug called early the next morning. "I'm really weak. I had diarrhea, and they're testing me for a bacteria."

"Oh no!"

"I'm trying to eat in spite of how I feel. I don't want to get weaker. I'll let you know about the results later this afternoon. I don't feel like talking. Bye."

That evening he was feeling better. We had a nice long talk on the phone. "The doctor put me on an anti-nausea regime that settled my stomach. I feel stronger."

I still had a scratchy throat the next morning and didn't want to expose Doug or the other patients. At this point I hoped it was only an allergy.

Jill delivered a care package including a frozen Costco hamburger and Jimmy John's chips for Doug's supper that night. She stopped by to see me on her way home. "Doug looked really good. He said he's been working out on his step stool and bike. He told me his white blood count was dropping as expected. There was a big drop today. Not sure what that means, but he said you would be happy to hear about it."

"I don't know what it means either except that the values have to drop and then go up. His declining counts have to do with Doug's cells dying off, and the donor cells growing up to take over. I'm not sure what determines when he can go home this time. I'll ask some questions when I go in tomorrow. During his last hospital stay, I could make more sense of it. Back then, we prayed every day his levels would go up." I shook my head and gestured to the couch. "Can you stay a minute?"

"I'd better get home to the kids."

ϵϵϵ

The next day, I flopped on the bed in Doug's bedroom and considered all I needed to do.

The phone rang. "Hi, it's Susan. How are things going?"

"Well," I cleared my throat. "You may regret calling."

"Oh gosh. What's wrong?"

"Nothing. I didn't mean to alarm you. Doug's fine. In fact, it's time to get the house ready for him to come home. I've been thinking of putting you to work."

"Wonderful! How can I help? Carole is in too."

"It's hard to ask, but I know your offers to help are sincere and well—I need you."

"Tell me what, where, and when. I'll call Carole."

"You'll never know how much this means to me. I've been distraught just thinking about everything I need to do."

The next morning Susan and Carole came over to help me clean the spaces where Doug would spend most of his time. They went crazy in his bedroom. An old-fashioned spring-cleaning like my mom used to do. I laundered the curtains. They took the blinds outside to scour and hose them until they were like new.

They scrubbed the walls and woodwork, Windexed the windows, and vacuumed everything in sight, including the lampshades. There was nary a dust bunny anywhere, even in Doug's closet. The weather cooperated. The hot sun quickly dried all the things we washed from vent covers to blinds to basket liners.

We moved most of the dust catchers from his room and hosed off all washable decorations that remained. Beth would have been proud. By the time we took a break for lunch, his bedroom was cleaner than it had ever been or ever will be again.

The work went quickly. It was actually fun to do with friends. I can't imagine how I'll ever repay them. I was able to go back and be with Doug that afternoon knowing the house was ready for his homecoming.

A few days later, I came home from the hospital to pick up the mail and get clean clothes for us both. I pulled into the driveway and saw Becky's car. I smelled paint as I walked through the house. "Becky? What's up?"

"Sarah and I are painting Doug's bathroom. I hope this is the right color. It's really bright. You said Crisp Green, right?"

"Oh you guys, thank you so much." I peered into the bathroom. "Yup, that's right. Good thing it'll be hidden away in Doug's small bathroom. It's his favorite color. He'd have it in the family room if I'd let him."

Becky smiled and Sarah laughed.

"I didn't know you were going to do this today. It's so awesome."

"We're happy to do it, Nonna." Sarah said.

"I'd help, but I need to head back to the hospital as soon as I pick up a few things."

Becky put her paintbrush down and gave me a hug. "No problem. Where would we put you? Sarah and I barely fit. This is a tiny bathroom. We'll be done in no time."

"I'm not going to tell Doug. I'll let it be his homecoming surprise. Thanks so much."

I loaded my car with the mail, snacks, and clean clothes. As I pulled out of the drive, tears welled in my eyes. I thanked God for prompting me to surrender my pride and recognize I needed help. My worries were such time-wasters. Things always got done somehow, often in ways I could never have imagined.

Sometimes I forget how much bigger God's radar screen is than my puny possibilities. One of the greatest blessings on this journey came from the magnitude of caring shown by so many.

Waiting to Go Home

On the way to the hospital, my mind focused on the remaining things I needed to do. Though the date of Doug's homecoming was uncertain, it was getting close. It was time to review the rules and discuss them with Doug in earnest.

I thought back to several weeks before Doug went into the hospital the first time. We had attended a class in preparation for the transplant. After a little more than an hour, Doug stood up loudly proclaiming he was hungry and left the room. Even in his hospital room, we argued about the rules. "Doug, please don't put your shoes up on the recliner. The nurse told you not to pick up trash off the floor. Keep your toothbrush away from mine."

Doug gave me lots of eye rolling and noncompliance. Until now, I left the intimidating binder at home and only talked to Doug about it in snippets. He just wasn't as focused as I was. I felt responsible for his safety at home and worried how I could pull it off without the structure of the hospital and support of the nurses and doctors. I was going to have to figure out how to make him give the rules proper attention. Though prepared to do battle, I hoped to avoid being Attila the Hun, so our marriage could remain intact.

€€€

The next day I went home to catch up on laundry and mail. The four-inch thick binder lay on the kitchen table and stared me in the face. It was time put it to use. As I flipped through the pages, Nurse Beth's words echoed: "Doug could do clean jobs not dirty jobs. No outside food from well-meaning friends. The kitchen table, stove, and sink must be kept clean with antiseptic wipes. Stay away from anyone who might be ill. Keep vehicles clean and the windows up."

Time to take the binder to the hospital. After I greeted Doug, I plopped it on his tray table. "Okay, honey, let's go over this stuff. You'll be going home soon." He ignored the first sentence and jumped on the second one.

"I can't wait. Jean will be glad to have me back. She's done a great job, but I know plenty of stuff will have fallen through the cracks."

"What? You're not going into work. I nearly killed myself and half our family and friends making the house clean enough for you. Your office will be impossible to get ready for you to be safe there. That place is full of mold from all the roof leaks and the inventory is dirty. I can imagine all the germs and other scary stuff lurking there to make you sick. Please tell me you're joking."

"We'll see how I feel. I can wear a mask and gloves."

"You have to agree to work from home at least for a few weeks."

"Don't worry about it now." He walked into the hall.

With great restraint, I let him go. After thirty minutes, he returned. I was ready for him.

"Okay, from the binder—if loading the dishwasher is a dirty job, surely you can see how taking out the garbage is a dirty job. So is wiping up the kitchen floor or cleaning a bathroom. It's second nature to you, but please stick to the rules." I nagged.

"I'll be fine. I just need to get home."

I shook my head and wondered how either one of us would survive.

ЄЄЄ

All Doug could think about was his homecoming. He was so done with the confinement of the small BMT department with all the med side effects and poking and prodding he endured. By this time, he couldn't bear to eat hospital food. He was still neutropenic and would be until at least the end of the hundred days. I brought him frozen dinners and appropriate treats to ease his frustration.

The days passed quickly for me but not for Doug. Every day, I reminded him to tear off a loop from each of his 100 link paper chains. He had two chains because when sisters, Emily and Samantha, heard Papa's magic number; they got busy making a colorful paper chain. Their cousins, Chelsea, Emma, and Jacob thought it was a great idea and fashioned their own 100 loops to help Papa count down the days. They couldn't wait until they would be able to play with Papa again.

Doug continued to have up and down blood values. His energy level and appetite waxed and waned. We hung on through fevers and chills. IV fluids were required again because Doug was unable to drink or eat enough. He was back on anti-nausea meds.

Clumps of hair littered his pillow. We secretly hoped he would beat the odds and keep his locks. He had kept them much longer than most chemo patients. But his time was coming.

The morning after Doug had a lethargic evening and a restless night, I went downstairs to the coffee shop and called Linda. "The doctors say Doug is doing well. He'll probably go home within days."

"Wonderful news! I'm so happy for you."

"Except he's feeling terrible—fevers, chills, nausea, and fatigue. I don't see how he can possibly go home. I'm scared to care for him alone with all these problems."

"Try to trust the doctors. They'll do what's best for Doug."

We discussed our families for a while. "I'd better get back upstairs."

"You guys hang in there. I pray for you both every day."

"Thanks, it makes all the difference."

I walked into Doug's room and did a double take. Doug was a new man, sitting up talking to the doctor.

"I was just telling Doug, it looks like he has turned the corner. His counts are edging up very slightly. He may and I stress *may* be able to go home tomorrow." Doctor Aljitawi pointed his finger at me. "If not it'll be Monday."

"What? How is that possible? He's been feeling terrible."

Doug shot me a dirty look.

"My guess is he'll probably be here through the weekend and leave Monday. He's actually doing very well. I'll see you tomorrow."

After the doctor left, I sat on the bed next to Doug. "I can't believe you could be that close to going home. You've been feeling terrible."

"Stop! Don't say anything negative. I'm going home. That's all that matters." He clicked on the TV. My cue to leave him alone and get myself together.

I grabbed my laptop and went to the snack room. After some chocolate chip cookies and a quick check of my emails, I was ready to go back to his room and behave.

When I returned, he was bald.

"A nurse came in and noticed all the hair on my pillow. She said it would be better to shave it rather than deal with the mess. I said, 'Let's do it.' It's not too bad is it?"

"Of course not." I tried to hide my shock. It was a weird milestone for me, but he seemed okay with it. "Anyway, you usually wear a baseball cap and I like that look."

"I'm going to take a shower and get this hair off me. Then I'll shave and feel human again."

And I'll work on getting used to the new hairdo.

Father's Day

On the morning of June 15, Doctor Aljitawi came into the room. "Good morning." He scanned Doug's chart. "Your platelets are up so you can exercise. Remember—you need to rest if you don't feel up to it."

"What about that magic ANC number?" I asked. (Absolute Neutrophil Count is a measure of a certain type of white blood cells that fight infection.)

"Actually, it has dropped."

All the air in my lungs escaped. I sank in my chair.

"We like to give the stem cells time to do their thing on their own, but sometimes they need a little jump start. It's the same medicine we give the donors to increase their production of stem cells. If the shot increases the counts satisfactorily, you can go home tomorrow."

Doug's eyes popped open wide. "Really? After all the ups and downs of the last few days, I can barely believe it! Thanks Doc." They shook hands.

I'm not sure whose smile was bigger, the doctor's or Doug's. Of course, I started tearing up.

"Remember, you'll be going to the clinic daily for the first week or so. They'll keep a close watch on you."

"That'll keep my blood pressure down," I said.

"Sounds good to me. I'll go twice a day if it gets me out of here," Doug said.

The doctor chuckled. "Depending on how you're doing, the frequency will decrease to two to three times weekly, then down to once a week for quite a while. I can't give you a prediction on how quickly that will happen, but you've been an amazing patient. I suspect you'll continue to progress well."

Later that day, they gave Doug a shot in the stomach. He smiled through the sting. We prayed it would be the magic bullet.

He continued to be lethargic off and on that day, but the chills and fevers appeared to be over.

On Sunday, June 16th, Doctor Aljitawi breezed into the room, all smiles. "Congratulations! The medicine did the trick. Once the paperwork is finished, you're free to go home. Be sure to take note of your appointment at the clinic for tomorrow. Happy Father's Day."

"I can't thank you enough for your professional skills and especially your caring and concern. You've been a real guardian angel for us," I said.

"I'll see you again. Most of the time I see patients in the hospital and quite a bit of my time is devoted to research, but I also keep in touch with outpatients at the clinic."

It was another easy date to remember. The first time Doctor Aljitawi sent Doug home for his two-week respite was his birthday. Now on Father's Day, he would finally go home to stay. He didn't beat the record of twelve days, but he was close. It was eighteen days after transplant, remarkable after the previous nerve-wracking week.

We gathered all our belongings from our twenty-three day stay. I was grateful Matt, our son-in-law, had taken the stationary bike home the day before. We could manage the rest. I made several hurried trips to the car while the nurse completed discharge details. I didn't want to test Doug's patience.

On our final trip out of Room 4109, Doug sat in a wheelchair loaded down with bags and miscellaneous supplies. It seemed as if we were moving in slow motion.

The nurses all looked up from their work and waved. "Good-bye and good luck you two. Doug, you were quite the memorable patient. We'll miss you."

"We'll miss you too." I croaked out past the lump in my throat. "Thank you so much for everything." My heart ached as if I was saying good-bye to family.

Doug waved, thanked them, and made a few final wisecracks. But I could see on his face, he was feeling emotional too. We were sure we would never be back there again. I was happy to be entering that annoying air lock room for the last time, and grateful I wasn't alone this time.

€€€

Loaded down like a couple of pack mules during the Gold Rush, Doug and I walked up the steps to our home. Juggling his bags, Doug unlocked the door and held it open for me. In the entryway, I dropped my bags and pushed them out of the way. I turned to see his reaction.

He flashed a grin, dropped his burden, and hugged me tightly. "I'm really here! For good! No more prison!" He peered into the family room. "You put my stationary bike in there?" He climbed on it and peddled. "Thanks."

"Yeah, I didn't want you to have to go downstairs. You can watch TV and ride to your heart's content."

"Where's the rug?"

"Emily and Chelsea helped me take it to the basement. I can keep the hardwood floor a lot cleaner. We'll get a new rug after your 100 days."

He dismounted. "I'm going to put my stuff away. Then we can have lunch at our very own kitchen table." He walked down the hall toward his bedroom.

I went into the kitchen to put away the snacks we'd brought home and start lunch. Then I heard Doug yell.

"Wow! My bathroom is Crisp Green. It looks incredible." Doug marched up to me. "When did you do that?"

"Becky and Sarah surprised me. So glad you like it. I found that crazy crisp green and bright blue shower curtain at Target, probably the only one on the planet that matches the walls."

"It looks awesome. Thanks a lot."

A Reason, A Season, or A Lifetime

People come into our lives for a reason, a season or a lifetime. I'm infinitely grateful to the anonymous writer who shared his or her wisdom. Those words helped me recognize answered prayers. Often earth angels came unbidden just when I needed them most.

Throughout our journey, I encountered many who came for each of those time-periods. The parking lot attendant who put his arm around me and told me it would be okay when I was frantic with worry. A patient sitting on a bench outside the hospital with whom I shared stories. She offered to pray for Doug and me. The woman who distracted me with a compliment that turned into a conversation during Doug's first bone marrow biopsy. The doctors, nurses and other medical staff who have been there for us. Some for a reason, some for a season, and some for a lifetime. Thankfully, the Locker Room Angels are here for the latter.

Some people came for a short season but influenced me for a lifetime. Doctor Wasserman was such a man. After we received Doug's diagnosis of leukemia and his need for a bone marrow transplant, word spread quickly. Friends expressed their concern and curiosity about the process.

I was reminded what a small world we live in during a conversation with Monte, a friend since college days.

"Did you say Doug has to have a bone marrow transplant, and he goes to University of Kansas Hospital?"

"Yup, that's the only way to save him from leukemia. It's the best hospital in the region. Thank God it's so close."

"There's a guy in my neighborhood who needs a bone marrow transplant. He goes there too. His name is Gary Wasserman. He's a doctor. Have you met him?"

"I don't think so."

"He's an amazing guy. He writes emails to the neighborhood about how he's doing—very interesting. I'll forward them if you want."

"That would be great. Thanks."

Monte walked to the door, then turned back. "Good luck to you and Doug. Keep me posted."

The next Sunday in church, a good friend mentioned Doctor Wasserman. She also lived in his neighborhood and was impressed with his writings. She wanted to be sure we had access to this remarkable man's inspiring emails.

One day while Doug was in Unit 41 getting chemo to prepare him for his transplant, I stepped into the hallway to call my son. After I hung up, a man about my age came up to me.

"How's your husband doing?"

"Pretty well. Thanks for asking. He's tired today."

"Several of the other patients and I have been discussing him. He's our hope, our benchmark. We see how much he exercises, and he seems to have a wonderful attitude. If he's doing well, maybe this isn't so bad and we can manage it too."

I nodded my head. "My husband's incredibly tough." I wanted to shake the man's hand, but that's a huge no-no in the germ-free Bone Marrow Transplant world. "My name is Evie. I'll be sure to let him know he's inspiring his fellow patients. He'll love that."

"Very nice to meet you. Everyone calls me Wass. Do you have a few minutes?"

"Sure. Doug's asleep. It'll be lovely to chat with someone. Visitors are scarce."

Wass grinned and nodded his head as we walked over to lean against the windowsill.

"After all Doug's been through, the big day is almost here. He gets his cells on May 29th.

"That's wonderful. I finally get my transplant in early June."

We talked about Doug for a bit. Then this charismatic man told me his story. KU had a difficult time trying to find him a donor. Finally, they located one in Germany. Just like Doug, he was unable to have the transplant as scheduled because of complications.

"By the time I was ready, the donor had backed out." He said this with no hint of anger or resentment.

"Oh my gosh!" I covered my face with my hands. "You must have been devastated. I can't imagine."

"That's behind me now. I waited several months. Finally, KU found a donor. I'm ready to start a whole new life. I just got married, and I adopted my wife's daughter, Madison, right after the wedding. She's the best thing that ever happened to me, next to her mother." He glanced at his watch. "Would you like to meet her? She'll be visiting any minute, but we can only see her through the window. She's seven. You know the rules."

"Oh yes, I know the rules. Most of our grandchildren are under twelve. I would love to meet her."

He turned toward the place she would be. "There she is! Isn't she beautiful?" We walked over to the window to see her smiling, waving, and blowing kisses. His face radiated joy. His positive attitude told me he would make it out of here to begin his new life.

After Madison left, we continued our conversation. After about five minutes, I blurted, "Oh my goodness! I know who you are. You live less than three miles from us in Independence. We have mutual friends. They've been forwarding your emails. I've enjoyed reading them. They inspire me."

His smile lifted my heart. "Thank you very much."

I didn't see Doctor Wass much after that. I assumed he was feeling worse, like Doug, because of the chemo required prior to transplant. The quiet hall testified to the patients' needs to rest in their rooms while they coped with nausea, exhaustion, and weakness. Stem cell recipients needed every ounce of energy they could muster to deal with the prelude to the big event. Cell Day for most of the unit drew close. The nurses placed decorated signs on their doors to announce that important date.

€€€

After we left the hospital, I followed Wass's emails. They were funny and uplifting, always full of fight, love, and hope. He was open to anything, even experimental drugs. KU BMT doctors tried everything until there was nothing more to do. His last email reduced me to heartbroken sobs.

One day in March 2014, he wrote. "I have accepted that I am at the end of my journey. This is not the same as quitting. I now understand the expression, 'My spirit is strong, but the flesh is weak.'" During his last days, he planned his own celebration of life event.

I later contacted his widow, Cheryl Wasserman, and learned what an extraordinary man had come into my life for that short season. Cheryl met me at Starbucks, and we visited as if we were old friends. She shared three beautiful memory books she had compiled. "Would it help to take these home while you write your chapter about Wass?"

"I would love to. Are you sure you want to let them out of your hands?"

"Sure, go ahead and take them."

"I'll return them as soon as I'm done. Thank you so much."

€€€

During our second meeting, I returned those treasures to her. We vowed to keep in touch. Perhaps Wass has given me the gift of a friend for a season or even a lifetime.

Doctor Wasserman was a beloved leader, educator, and physician at Children's Mercy where he had a 41-year career. All who knew him respected and loved him. He received many awards and certificates for his outstanding career. The Children's Mercy Hospital ER waiting room was dedicated to him on December 19, 2013: The Gary "Doc Wass" Wasserman Waiting Room.

Even with a transplant, Wass couldn't beat his leukemia. Maybe it was because he had an additional underlying blood problem that had plagued him since his twenties. Doctors back then hadn't expected him to live longer than ten years. He lived a life full of joy, travel, and service for many years beyond that. Cheryl said every birthday was a huge celebration for him.

I wish his story had ended differently. It was difficult to lose this man whom I had met only for a season. But he will be remembered for a lifetime—not just by me, but by the many lives he touched. I will always be inspired by his positive spirit, willingness to fight, friendliness, good humor, and the joy he brought wherever he went.

I added him to my list of angels.

Early Days at Home

Our daily visits to the clinic didn't last long. Doug was doing well and after the first week, his doctor declared him ready for twice weekly. He tolerated his pill breakfast well. His daily meds included tacrolimus—the anti-rejection med. Tac levels, as we came to call them, were checked each time we went to the clinic as part of the long list of other indicators that told the doctors how Doug was doing. I never realized how much our blood reveals about the condition of our bodies. His tacrolimus level was always good, but that med depleted his magnesium, typical for many patients. Magnesium is important for muscle and nerve function, blood sugar levels, blood pressure, and making protein, bone, and DNA. Especially in the beginning of treatment, the oral form of this nutrient wasn't potent enough to keep up with the loss that tacrolimus created. Doug hated the procedure because it was a slow IV drip. It often took a couple of hours.

"I tolerate this stuff well. Please run it quicker so I can get out of here."

Some of the nurses heeded his begging and ran it quicker, checking often to make sure he was handling it okay.

Doug found a kindred spirit in one of the clinic's male nurses. "I hope I get Jordan today. I'll get out of here in no time."

"Hey man, how ya doing? Did you hear the one about...? Jordan quickly became a friend and always had a shady joke. He ran the IV as rapidly as he could while keeping Doug safe from reactions to the magnesium.

When Jordan took care of Doug's treatment, I left to walk the halls or get something from the cafeteria. I was happy to let those two talk their boy talk. My husband was in good hands. He was always smiling or laughing when I walked back into the room.

ƐƐƐ

During the rest of the 100 days, Doug had to have someone with him at all times. As an independent guy, he not only resented this rule, but thought it was ridiculous.

One day I went outside to weed the garden for a few minutes. Our neighbor, Ted, came to the fence to ask about Doug. We visited longer than I realized. Suddenly, I had a sinking feeling and ran back to the house. I threw the screen door open and saw Doug on the floor in the kitchen. He was sweating and weak.

"Oh gosh! What happened? I knelt by him.

"I don't know. Suddenly I was weak and dizzy. I started sweating, and I couldn't stand. I was trying to call you."

"I didn't mean to be out there so long, but I never expected this. Did you hurt yourself?"

"No. I just slumped to the floor."

I helped him to the couch. "I'll get a cold washcloth and call the clinic."

In a few minutes, Doug sat up looking much better. "It's the new med they gave me. Don't ask me why I think that, I just do."

I put my finger to my lips to shush him. "Hang on. I'm talking to the clinic." After a few minutes, I hung up the phone. "The nurse said to bring you right in. Do you think you can get to the car or should I see if Ted can help you?"

"I can make it. I feel better."

I drove to the clinic as fast as I dared.

The nurse took us into an exam room.

Doctor Ganguly came in shortly. "What's going on? I hear you nearly passed out."

"I believe I've had a reaction to a new med." Doug told him which one.

120

"It's possible with that medication. We've prescribed it prophylactically so let's discontinue it and see how you feel."

How in the world Doug knew that pill was the reason for his episode, I'll never know, but apparently, he was right.

€€€

I vowed never to leave him for more than ten minutes. It continued to make him crazy. Since he couldn't stay home alone and hated the idea of having babysitters, he drove me to do errands. He liked the idea of getting out of the house but had to wait in his van while I rushed in to grab what we needed. I worried about him even with the air conditioning going. He'd search for a shady spot and read a book. That summer was very hot, and it was difficult to find any place out of the sun.

One day he drove me to the grocery store, dropped me off, and went to find a parking spot. I waited to see where he parked then raced through my lengthy list. In the long checkout line, I huffed, and puffed and tapped my toe. Finally, I hustled from the store. The van wasn't where I expected it to be.

I darted around the parking lot, pushing my loaded cart. Doug was nowhere. My t-shirt was soaked from worry and the relentless sun. Did he suffer a heat stroke and someone took him to the hospital? Tears flooded my cheeks. I was so upset, it never occurred to me to call him. Looking back, I realize how irrational I was. Did he drive to the hospital? Should I call 9-1-1? Where could he possibly be?

Sanity returned, and I called his cell. I sobbed, "Where are you? What happened?"

"For Pete's sake! I drove the five blocks home. I had to go to the bathroom. You would've gone nuts if I came into the store to use the restroom. Why are you crying?"

"I didn't know what happened. You were gone."

"Calm down. We can't live like this. What did you think happened?"

"You're right. I seem to go straight to the worst."

"I'll be right there."

"Sorry."

εεε

I gradually calmed down. It was the only way to survive. Phone calls to Jean at work were soon not enough for Doug.

"I'm going to check in at work for just for a few minutes. I'll wear a mask and gloves."

"Please call me when you get there."

Jean, his office wife, would do all she could to take care of him and send him home as soon as possible. There was nothing else to do. I couldn't tie him to a chair.

Our Second and Third Homes

Our previous stomping grounds included Independence, Blue Springs, and Lees Summit, Missouri. Doug's leukemia, bone marrow transplant and subsequent treatments created a new home for us on the Kansas side. Located west of the Plaza, the University of Kansas Cancer Center—Westwood became our second home. It was the place I ran to when anything went wrong with Doug. If I could just get him there, we were safe. The doctors, nurses and other staff knew us well, and they knew exactly what to do.

We spent many hours there for routine exams and treatments, but panicked weekends made it truly our home. "Doug isn't doing well. I don't know what's wrong but he's lethargic and weak," I croaked into the phone, my heart racing.

"Come right on in. We'll be waiting for you. Come through the limited access door in case Doug is contagious."

I loaded Doug into the car, sometimes with the help of a neighbor or family member. The thirty-minute drive seemed endless, but relief was at the end.

As we approached the parking garage, Doug rallied. Except for a couple of occasions, he refused to let me push him in a wheelchair. We parked the car, and I bit my tongue as I watched him struggle to the elevator.

We rode up to the third floor and entered the limited access door. I grabbed an ever-present tissue from the counter as tears of relief spilled from my eyes. We were safe.

A nurse approached with concern in her eyes. "Come on Doug. Let's get you into a room. What's going on?"

They would soon figure it out. Most of the time, they gave him what he needed, and our misery ended there. After a couple of hours of treatment, we were free to return home.

Sometimes his condition required more serious intervention. They had to send Doug for in-patient care. Even then, the clinic staff went the second mile. They fast-tracked the arrangements so we could go directly to the fourth floor of KU hospital. No emergency room or admission department hassle to cause further stress. The hospital nurses quickly prepared a room for Doug. By the time we arrived, they were ready and immediately busied themselves with his care.

Sometimes we had a room in Unit 41 BMT—the place we thought was in our past. We were surprised to see how it had expanded since Doug's transplant. Unfortunately, the need for transplants had grown rapidly. When the BMT unit was full, they would take us across the hall to Unit 42. KU's fourth floor became our third home, but thankfully not often.

Doug says every day he's not in the hospital is a good day. I agree, but I'm so grateful for our second and third homes. Doug receives treatments there that keep him going. Those brilliant caring physicians continually look for medications and treatments that will make Doug's life longer and better.

Lessons on the Journey

The most valuable message I learned was not to limit myself. God gifts me with whatever it takes to do what must be done.

My senior year in high school, I toyed with the idea of going into the medical field. My best friend was going to be a nurse, and she had the temperament. As we discussed my problem with panicking and fainting at the sight of blood and/or people in pain, we decided it was too much for me to overcome. I crossed nursing off my list and stayed as far away from hospitals and doctors as possible.

I was lucky to raise four children with few medical emergencies. Life threw me a horrendous curve when Doug got sick. The forced transition from squeamishness to caring for PICC lines, bloody wounds, administering shots, and being strong as my husband suffered in so many ways was a miracle. I stood by him all alone through circumstances that nearly killed him—situations where my strongest urge was to run from the room and hide somewhere far away.

Dazed, I sat in small windowless sterile rooms while nurses prepped Doug for the next horrendous procedure. My presence there was incomprehensible, and the outside world felt far away. The calm and good cheer of the nurses kept me sane.

I watched as they accessed his jugular vein with a large tube. My world began to spin. Somehow, Doug was often on his best behavior in those situations. He cracked jokes or interviewed the nurses, keeping things semi-normal in circumstances that were surreal and kaleidoscopic for me. "Where are you from? Do you have a family? Why did you choose nursing?"

Really Doug? Who cares? They are about to invade your body in an effort to save your life. His ability to rise above the circumstances had to be a gift from God. His demeanor saved me from swooning off my chair and landing on the floor. Clearly from his vantage point, he could not see what I saw, and he must not have completely understood his circumstances.

One time, when his hemoglobin continued to drop despite daily transfusions, Doctor Ganguly, a pharmacist and a research physician stood in Doug's room. They were determined to save him. They hooked him up to a huge machine that sounded like a rickety airplane trying to take off. His blood had to run through this monstrosity to be cleansed of the agent that was causing the deterioration.

When he felt better, Doug thanked Doctor Ganguly for saving his life.

The doctor's response? He raised his eyes and pointed to the ceiling with a smile. "I only did my job. He did the rest."

That incident was only one of many I acknowledged were serious beyond my understanding. I recognized it was not in me to survive all of this. God blessed me with courage and faith, perhaps even a sense of oblivion at times.

Let the record show Doug was sometimes the worst patient ever. I felt as if I had to explain his failed humor or even his rudeness. He acted large and in charge on many occasions and made some ugly first impressions.

When he realized his anxiety, pain, or fear had made him incorrigible, he apologized. Eventually, he put on his salesman's hat and his charming personality won over nearly everyone who took care of him. I learned to trust in that.

Many people quote the conventional wisdom, "Live one day at a time." In truth, it's impossible to live even more than one moment at a time. That lesson has been hammered home. Utmost joy and horrendous fear must be lived in the present.

A planner by nature, to-do lists filled my Franklin planner, and overflowed my purse. I had never been open to accepting changes without a fuss.

Our journey profoundly altered that pattern. I still write lists but know they are only temporarily valid. Flexibility and owning lack of control are the only ways to keep my life livable.

I learned that compassionate strangers offered smiles and kind words. From the parking lot attendants to doctors and nurses, to those who took care of the equipment, cleaned Doug's room, or took his vitals—these people blessed us with kindness beyond what we imagined.

I met patients and their family members who touched me with their concern, faith and caring. Within that unique community, we shared many prayers and hopes for and with each other.

When life teeters on the edge of death, it's easy to drop any pretense and bare your soul to those who understand best. We shared the mystery and uncertainty that robbed the ordinary and the trivial from our lives. Together, we stared down a path that may or may not include the loved ones who fought this battle against cancer. Would we have to leave the hospital without them?

The things we worry about are often taken care of much easier than we expect. My worries about how I would get the house clean enough for Doug vanished when friends and family came to the rescue. Jeanne made it possible to get the stationary bike to Doug. Matt took it home. How would the donor cells be ready at just the right time? They were sent to the hospital and kept frozen. The list was long, and I felt very blessed.

Most of all, I learned that angels come in all shapes and sizes. They exist all around us, often in the most unlikely places. Now I look for them and fully expect to find them. They rarely descend from heaven wearing white robes, halos above their heads and glittery wings on their backs.

Sometimes they wear white lab coats, stethoscopes around their necks, and show off data entry skills as they order new meds and treatments on a computer.

Now and then, they burst from locker rooms wearing smelly hockey jerseys, ice skates and carrying hockey sticks.

Epilogue

Our four-year-old grandson, Otto, who thinks Papa hung the moon, used only seven words to nail Doug's physical condition better than any doctor. He said, "Papa, your whole body is an owie." Five years after the bone marrow transplant that saved his life, my husband struggles with chronic Graft versus Host Disease.

It has attacked his skin in a dramatic way. He has weird lesions on his feet—a catchall word used because no one knows exactly what they are. We do know they hurt and refuse to heal. Doug describes the pain as walking with sharp rocks in his shoes. No surprise, he refuses to use a walker or a cane.

Skin cancer surgeries are an ongoing trial. His left—dominant hand—suffered a deep wound that required a skin graft after Mohs surgery. This procedure involves a precise surgical technique, which progressively removes thin layers of skin. Lab experts examine the tissue in an onsite lab. The surgeon continues to remove layers until the sample returns free of cancer. The healing process has been ongoing for endless months as the tissue fights to granulate (fill in and heal). Doug's hand is swollen and sore. It resembles what I imagine leprosy to look like. At one point, he had a bad infection in the wound. It took us back to the hospital for complicated diagnosis and the right antibiotic.

After that episode, we took on home infusion to continue antibiotic treatment. Doug wore a pump night and day. Showers and sleeping were complicated. It took us a while to figure out how to ready the new dose of medication each day. In the beginning, tubing and battery changes kept us confused and frustrated. The nurse who taught us the procedure gave us a 24-hour hotline. We used it often and gratefully for the first few days.

The left side of Doug's neck and face are tight, red, and itchy in several areas where basal cell and squamous cell carcinomas were removed. A cautionary tale that prolonged sun exposure can cause harm through the window of a car when you spend lots of time behind the wheel. Tests show glass blocks UVB, which causes sunburn. Since only windshields are treated to block UVA, a car's side windows allow it to penetrate.

Doug has grappled with the effective but high anxiety Mohs method multiple times. We joined a dozen patients and caregivers to wait in a comfortable waiting room full of snacks and beverages, hoping and praying the results would indicate all cancer was gone the first time. If not, the doctor would remove another layer and send it to the lab for examination until the tissue was cancer-free.

While I waited for Doug to get out of surgery, I glanced discreetly around the room at all the patients. Bandages covered arms, hands, cheeks, noses, eyelids, lips, and ears. I wondered why cancer had attacked each particular area.

I prayed each patient would hear his/her name called, followed by, "You're all done today." On occasion, Doug had to wait two and three times to hear those words. We are vigilant about checking for sores that don't heal or appear to heal and come back, especially when they bleed. It's difficult to discern what is GVHD and what cancer is. Doug often has biopsies to make sure. We've learned the hard way that getting skin cancer removed early makes Mohs much less miserable.

Doug has scleroderma, a rare, self-limiting skin condition defined by progressive thickening and hardening of the skin, usually on the areas of the upper back, neck, shoulders, and face. Unfortunately, for Doug, it is not limited to those areas. It has attacked his trunk, arms and legs. His abdomen is as hard as a tree trunk. A punch to his stomach would result in the perpetrator hurting his/her hand.

That tightness affects his ability to expand his lungs. Pulmonary function tests show an alarming decrease in his once healthy lung capacity. The doctor noted Doug's original 125% of expected capacity has mitigated the effect.

Scleroderma mottles and dries the skin, creating redness, itching, and tightness that are untouched by the lotions and potions Doug tries endlessly. We have a better supply of wound care products, anti-itch lotions, anti-pain ointments and other skin care merchandise than Walgreens.

Doug has a strange hole in his stomach, which tunnels beneath the skin. As prescribed by wound care specialists, I pack the wound with packing strips and medicines daily. The procedure seems to be helping the cavern heal, but oh so slowly.

Chronic GVHD and/or chemo have affected Doug's teeth. He has lost at least ten teeth, which makes it difficult for him to chew his food. His mouth is sensitive and some foods are too spicy or too crunchy. Fear of infection has delayed finding a solution.

Otto was right. "Papa's whole body is an owie."

Despite the challenges, Doug works every day, often fighting exhaustion as he waits for one of the good days. Whenever possible, he exercises like a maniac. He rides a stationary bike when it's too hot or cold. He often rides his bike for an hour outside in the early morning or late evening to avoid the sun. Stretching and weight-lifting are part of his daily routine unless he simply cannot manage it.

Flexibility reigns at our house. Plans can go by the wayside in less than an instant. We truly live one moment at a time. Some projects—such as my new kitchen—still shine in the future. They bring hope for a return to a healthy life, when Doug's condition improves enough to allow the remodel.

My heart breaks as I watch Doug struggle with pain and fatigue. Much of the time, my pleas for him to take it easy go unheeded. Though I worry he does too much, I'm proud of his strength and determination. Those qualities are what have kept me from losing him. The days he feels good fill us with gratitude and hope.

Grandchildren are our secret weapon. They give us love, laughter and provide us with inspiration and anecdotes.

Jacob, our nine-year-old grandson feels the same about Papa as Otto does. Whenever we sit down to eat with the family, he jockeys to sit by Doug, edging out his sisters and cousins. He hangs on every word Papa says from Doug's tall tales to advice on how to get six pack abs.

Jacob always has some new physical triumph to show Papa: increased pushups, higher wheelies on his bike or more air as he flips onto the couch. Sometimes he's excited to tell Papa he has shaved seconds off his Rubik Cube record.

"Watch this Papa" always precedes Jacob's new accomplishments. Doug and Jake are building a Ninja Warrior course in our basement. Pound for pound, Jake's small body is the strongest in the world—for sure in Papa and Jake's world.

All eleven grandkids love Papa with a love that keeps Doug going as much as the medications he must take daily. They ask about him, and I know they pray for him. Papa watches our little princesses, who used to dance around the living room with feather boas while he played his Conga drum transform into beautiful young women. Doug vows to be strong enough to provide bodyguard service for them.

Doctor Abhyankar is KU Cancer Clinic's chronic GVHD expert. He has been our primary physician for the last several years. His soft-spoken manner, compassion, and tenacity to stay on top of new meds and treatments fill us with confidence at every appointment. He never gives up on Doug. Doctor Abhyankar ensures that Doug gets the best treatment in the most efficient manner possible. Once when Doug was in crisis, Doctor Abhyankar gave me his cell phone number. (I discarded it immediately after that emergency to avoid temptation.)

One of the ongoing treatments Doug experiences two times a week every other week is extracorporeal photopheresis (ECP). This process provides the least side effects to help his body with chronic GVHD. Doug has a specialized port in his chest to facilitate this therapy. Leukocytes are collected from peripheral blood. They are exposed to a photosensitizing agent and treated with ultraviolet radiation. Then the blood is re-infused into Doug. The process takes almost two hours. The ECP department is a comfortable place for Doug. The staff is skillful at what they do. When they are not busy, they serve as expert conversationalists to pass the time when Doug is not dozing or reading. He often brings cookies to share.

Doug is an inspiration and a hope to all who know him. He brings hope into impossible circumstances. I expect he will continue to fight his battles and amaze his doctors, perhaps giving them fodder for research and medical journals.

Possibly even a continuing story for me to tell.

Doug's Story

Until I got on the ice with cancer, no one described me as a patient person. I liked to do things fast. In fact, on most hockey nights, I was the fastest guy on the ice—even at 62 years old! Our commissioner, Ric Lutz, introduced me to any new players as the old fast guy.

When I took on cancer, I learned to slow down and have patience.

At twenty-one, I set two goals for myself. I would play hockey until I was eighty-five, and I would live to 100. That plan was in jeopardy.

At one point during my stay in KU Hospital Room 4109, things looked especially grim. I received a unit of blood every day, but my hemoglobin still dropped. I thought I wasn't long for this world.

I asked Evie to bring me some writing paper. It was time for good-bye letters, and the divulging of my secret spaghetti sauce recipe. My eleven-year-old granddaughter, Emily, wanted my famous spaghetti at her wedding.

When you play hockey and compete against cancer, you gain some amazing teammates and coaches—people who are pulling for you and want you to succeed against all odds.

While the medicines and medical staff kept me from dying, they couldn't really save my life. I loved the life I had before cancer. My new life is entirely different, and not of my choosing.

My days are now full of struggles with cancer and chemo side effects, which may last the rest of my life. I might never play hockey again. But I'm full of gratitude for the Locker Room Angels and all my other teammates who continue to help me endure and survive.

Acknowledgements

First and foremost, I acknowledge my husband, who was a steadfast support throughout the long process of writing this memoir. His endless encouragement and willingness to let me tell the agonizing details of his struggle—even those times that were not flattering to him—were heroic.

From the bottom of our hearts, Doug and I thank Reed Ginn, a pharmacist, young husband and father, who took time out of his busy life to donate the life-saving stem cells that gave Doug a second chance at life.

I'm forever grateful to The Locker Room Angels, especially Ric Lutz, Bob Price and Roy Haler. They put together a fundraiser that started Doug's horrendous medical journey on a high note. No other group of supporters could accomplish this feat. Participation in The Doug Kalvelage Speed Tournament, from his teammates and those players who had never met Doug, represented a brotherhood that will always be huge in his life. Their shared love of hockey makes them treasured friends.

I'm grateful to family and friends who provided love, caring and strength even when they couldn't come to the hospital because of necessary restrictions posed by young children. I'm indebted to those who were able to come: Roy Haler, Becky Gorden, Susan Bresler, Matt Rogge, Jill Rogge, Jeanne Earnest, Allan and Sherry Rowett. Special kudos to those who visited from out-of-town: Kay Watnick, Ginny Hirata, Roz Kalvelage, Katey and Ron Calpo, and Jamie Harriman with our granddaughters Penelope and Amelia.

It's impossible to describe the connection we felt to those of you who wrote in the Guestbook of CaringBridge. We eagerly awaited those messages many times each day.

Special thanks to our grandchildren who grieved the loss of Papa's presence in their lives, some of them too young to understand what was wrong. They filled Papa's walls with artwork and love that made his claustrophobic room bearable.

Thanks to all who prayed for us. Some of our prayer warriors didn't even know us personally but prayed at the request of friends and family. The Rogge family and those on the prayer chain of Good Shepherd Community of Christ offered countless prayers. We felt the power of those prayers as they sustained our faith and brought miracles.

Linda Mai, my tireless writing buddy and critique partner deserves my gratitude from the beginning of the project through the end. She offered astute editing and comments always with kindness.

I'm in debt to the Kansas City Writers Guild (KCWG) for their years of considerate listening, encouragement and valuable critiquing.

The comments of beta readers: Jason Gorden, Sharon Bandlow, Kay Watnick, Jeanne Earnest and Gin Hirati made me believe my story was worthwhile.

I owe much to my friend and writing coach, Rebecca Thesman. She kept me on track and made my dream a reality.

Michael Freeman, Valiant Courier Publications, was a joy to work with and captured my vision for the cover art.

Sally Jadlow helped me with the mysteries of technology. My son, Jason, stepped in at the last minute when I was at the end of my rope. He completed the final formatting.

Thanks to Jean Palmer who worked with unfaltering devotion to keep KC Quality Products, Inc. alive and well so Doug would have a business to come back to.

I'm forever grateful to KU Medical Center and all its doctors, nurses, social workers and other medical staff, who went above and beyond in their caring and personal involvement with us.

Doctor Abhyankar continues to be a rock on our journey. The staff in the ECP department takes care of Doug with proficient expertise. They make the ongoing therapy bearable.

Doctor Sinclair, KU Clinic's palliative care doctor, has been a blessing as he helps us with the misery of GVHD side effects. He chats with Doug about their mutual interest—hockey—at every visit while they work together to find ways to help Doug get the best quality of life in spite of his chronic pain. Doctor Sinclair's kindness and compassion are remarkable. His staff is always available and ready to help us.

Finally, to my God, who was and is present with us in hospital waiting rooms, clinics, doctors' offices, and emergency rooms, through countless life-threatening episodes. Somehow, He infuses us with enough courage and faith to survive each moment.

He sat with me at the keyboard when I was discouraged and sent experts to help with the daunting process of getting my words into a real book.

About the Author

Evie Kalvelage lives in Independence, Missouri with her husband Doug. Her family includes two daughters, two daughters-in-law and one stepdaughter, as well as two sons and two sons-in-law.

She delights in being a grandma (Nonna) to eleven grandkids. They have been the subject of essays that appeared in Best Times, Wisconsin Women, and The Storyteller Magazine. She also writes stories for the Community of Christ blog, Daily Bread, and her congregational newsletter.

This is Evie's debut memoir. A journey that has taken her from being squeamish and frightened of the medical world to becoming a compassionate and able caregiver for her husband. She weaves faith, honesty, and humor together in a way that gives inspiration, reasons for gratitude and hope to those who fight battles with cancer.

Evie's favorite place on earth is a beach in Florida. She feels blessed to visit yearly for a one week writing retreat with her best friend.

She likes to read, knit, crochet, and spend time with grandchildren. She engages in activities such as pickleball, walks and bike rides. The grandkids' sporting and music events keep her entertained. Evie is blessed with a loving church family.

Doug and Evie hold onto hope that someday they will be able to travel, hike, golf and play tennis together again.

Made in the USA
Monee, IL
30 September 2022

14881312R00085